EVERY BREATH YOU TAKE

A Doctor's Guide to
Reducing Indoor Air Pollution

B.P. Loughridge, M.D.

Health Design, Inc.

Acknowledgments

I wish to express my heartfelt thanks and gratitude to my darling wife and three wonderful daughters who have made each breath I have taken much fresher and more vibrant than the previous breath.

And a special thanks to Carl H. Young, III and Rocks-DeHart Public Relations. Carl inspired me to write the book and Rocks-DeHart made it all come together.

Table of Contents

Introduction

How often do you think about the air you breathe? Probably not very often, though the mere fact that you've picked up this book shows you realize it's an important issue. The truth is, most of us don't pay much attention to air quality unless we're stuck in traffic behind a rattletrap belching forth noxious fumes, having a few drinks in a smoke-choked bar, or inspecting an old building for asbestos. My point is this: we don't spend much time worrying about the air in our homes, schools, and businesses.

It's very human to assume that because something is "familiar" it must also be harmless. The issue of air quality weighs on *my* mind only because my career has been based on helping people safeguard and improve their health. I am a cardiovascular surgeon, but more important, I am a vocal and persistent advocate of pursuing a healthy lifestyle. I consider it my mission to urge you to eat right, exercise regularly, drink lots of water, control the level of stress in your life ... and be aware of what you're breathing every day.

And you might be breathing some very bad stuff, indeed! The air in your home, your office, or your child's school could be filled with dust mites, mold spores, roach particles, pollen, pet dander, lead dust, radon gas, carbon monoxide, airborne viruses and bacteria, or any combination thereof. And these contaminants can make you very, very sick. If you are plagued with allergies or suffer from asthma, you probably already realize that bad air can pack a nasty wallop. If you're in perfect health, you've probably never given it a second thought—but the sobering truth is that if you don't take proactive measures today, you may not be so hale and hearty tomorrow!

My purpose in writing this book is not to frighten but to inform. I have always believed the old adage that knowledge is power. When you understand the factors that cause or exacerbate airborne contaminants, you empower yourself to take steps to change them! That's why *Every Breath You Take* is filled with solutions—solutions you can implement now to give yourself and your loved ones the gift of fresh, clean, healthy air.

I would be remiss if I did not put my words in the proper context. I am writing this introduction in early November of 2001. Even as I type these words, America is in the throes of a bioterrorism scare focused on inhalation anthrax. It is my fervent hope that by the time this book is published, we will have this deadly disease under control. Yet, I also hope we'll emerge from this crisis with a renewed concern for the safety of the very air that gives us life.

The more knowledge I obtain, the more I see the human body as a miracle. And the respiratory system is a critical part of it. You breathe in and out about 23,000 times a day, and you don't even have to think about it. That's a good thing, of course; if you had to concentrate on the body's mechanisms to make them work, you wouldn't be able to put food on the table, save the planet, create a soul-stirring painting, or read your kids a bedtime story. Still and all, it's important that we pause long enough in our daily activities to give some thought to the quality of the air we breathe every day.

Don't you agree? I believe that after you read *Every Breath You Take*, you will! As I reiterate throughout the book, ensuring that you and your loved ones are safe and healthy requires effort. You may have to wash the bedclothes more often, replace your carpet with hardwood floors, fix some leaky pipes, or install an air-filtration system. But when you consider the rewards of taking these relatively simple steps, you will have to admit that the payoff is worth the effort.

This book is the result of many years of research. I present it to you in the hope that it will improve your life. So take a deep breath and start reading. I wish you good luck and vibrant health on your journey toward clean, pure, livable air!

CHAPTER 1

Is Your Indoor Air Making You Sick?

Air, Air Everywhere

L ook around you. I mean really look around, right now, wherever you are sitting, standing, or working at this very instant. Take a moment … what do you see? You're probably in familiar surroundings—a room somewhere in a building, of course. You could be sitting at the counter in your kitchen or curled up in front of the fire in your den. You might be crammed in a claustrophobic office cubicle or sitting in a reception room waiting for an appointment. If I asked you to describe these surroundings, you'd probably tell me that you see some furniture, four walls, a window or two, another person maybe, and perhaps a stack of newspapers or even this morning's breakfast dishes lying in the sink.

The one thing you probably didn't think of adding to your description of your surroundings is the air that is all around you. Why? Because you can't see it, feel it, or probably even smell it. Air is invisible, and you probably aren't used to giving it very much thought. But what if I told you that the *most important* thing about the room you are in at this moment is the quality of its air?

Indoor Pollution Invades All Environments

We are all pretty well versed in the hazardous effects of puffing on a cigarette or even being in the vicinity of someone else who is smoking. A cigarette burning in an ashtray emits significant amounts of tar, carbon monoxide, hydrogen cyanide, and nicotine into the air. People unlucky enough to be near cigarette smoke end up breathing in these chemicals that, along with being exposed to these toxins, can result in allergic reactions as well as a slew of symptoms resulting from the body's natural defense mechanisms and stress reactions to this most offensive pollutant.

"But, Dr. Bill," you might say to me, "nobody is smoking in my house. They don't allow smokers at my place of work, and there's certainly no smoking in my kid's school. My air's all right ... isn't it?"

In a word: No. It isn't. Chances are that even if you are a most meticulous housekeeper, there is at least *some* dust floating about your home. You may be battling a roach problem—a nuisance that is found in even the finest and most pristine of palaces! Microscopic mold spores are making a home in those moist cracks and crevices you don't even notice, and pollen probably pervades your premises. You may have a pet that pollutes your environment, and you may even be living with lead, asbestos, or radon or be in danger of exposure to potentially deadly doses of carbon monoxide.

And there are new and frightening threats to the safety of our indoor air. These threats are sinister and evil because rather than coming from natural elements or being the direct result of our own lifestyle choices, they are perpetrated by criminals who intentionally spread their poisons with the expected result of doing us harm. Of course I am referring to the threat of bioterrorism and the spread of bacterial and viral contaminants such as anthrax and smallpox. While the recommendations I make in this book may not be able to completely shield you and your loved ones from the results of these diabolical acts, employing some of the air-cleaning techniques recommended in this book, such as utilizing an air-filtration system, can reduce the ability of airborne microscopic germs to spread and is at least one line of defense.

A New Breed of Illness Brought On by Your Air

Any one of the myriad pollutants that affects indoor air quality, and it is likely that you're living with a combination of them, can be the cause of undiagnosed and untreated illness in your family and you. For the past century or so, physicians have focused their diagnoses and treatments on illness caused by bacterial and viral infections, heart disease, and cancer. But in the past several years, health-care professionals have begun to recognize a new breed of illnesses linked to man-made and naturally occurring elements in the environment. Research shows that the majority of environmental illness such as asthma, Legionnaire's disease, and humidifier fever, along with building-related illness and hypersensitivity pneumonitis are the direct result of breathing unclean air in our homes, our workplaces, and our schools. In fact, over the last twenty-five years, a link has actually been made between polluted indoor air and such notorious killers as coronary heart disease, peripheral vascular arterial disease, and lung cancer.

Allergic responses to indoor pollutants—including fatigue; headaches; chronic cough; itchy, watery eyes; runny noses and sneezing; and wheezing and shortness of breath—are increasing. And the likely cause is the air we breathe!

Sick-Building Syndrome Is on the Rise

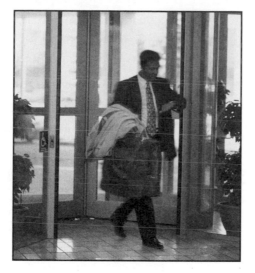

Beginning in the late 1960s and in the 1970s, construction experts decided to build homes and offices in a new way. The emphasis was on making buildings quieter and tighter—keeping noise and intruders out and, unfortunately, keeping fresh air from properly circulating as well! The result of this phenomenon is that we now have a new lexicon for describing illnesses that occur when toxins and allergens are re-circulated and not allowed to escape or be diluted with fresh air: *sick-building syndrome.*

Sick-building syndrome has come to describe a situation in which building occupants experience immediate, non-specific health effects after being exposed to some allergen within the building. These effects can include headaches, dizziness, sinus congestion, sneezing, eye and throat irritation, malaise, fatigue, and muscle aches that have no apparent cause.

Since indoor air pollution exists in every building or occupied structure, it is the degree of pollution that becomes the critical issue. Certain construction materials, paints, and finishes can produce symptoms of sick-building syndrome, as can toxins resulting from inadequate airflow and circulation. Inhabitants of sick buildings—office workers and students— end up breathing noxious harmful pollutants every day, and the effects can devastate their health! The only "cure" seems to be employing better airflow systems and, if possible, removing the toxic substances that may be adding to the problem.

Don't Despair—You *Can* Clean Your Air!!

"So, Dr. Bill," you might say with a sigh, "I guess we are all just doomed! We can't very well stop breathing, can we?"

No, we can't all stop breathing. And I'm not advocating that everyone run out and purchase gas masks and walk around in haz-mat suits! What you can do is follow the steps I have outlined in this book. Take charge of your indoor air by first and foremost learning where the likely contaminants are hiding and implementing a strategy to attack and destroy these enemies of clean air and good health. You can employ new and improved home-maintenance and house-cleaning techniques. You can keep your air safer by utilizing special air-filtration systems, and you can encourage your office manager, building superintendent, and school officials to do the same! The right air-filtering system can even serve as a first line of defense against the invasion of disease-causing and life-threatening germs.

Control Asthma Triggers: Clear Polluted Indoor Air

Asthma affects an estimated 150 million people worldwide. Asthma is a chronic, serious affliction of the lungs and occurs as the result of an inflammatory response by the lungs to allergens. And oftentimes these allergens are polluting your indoor air. If left unchecked and untreated, an asthma attack may be life threatening or even fatal. People with asthma must first and foremost obtain sound medical treatment. In addition, they should limit, if not eliminate, their exposure to asthma-producing allergens by utilizing environmental control measures such as utilizing a high efficiency, high filtration air cleaner in the bedroom and using surface cleaners that are bagless and incorporate a multi-level filter system that meets or exceeds HEPA standards.

Common Triggers for Asthma Attacks

INFECTIONS: Colds, other viruses, and bacterial infections can act as triggers by initiating the air passages. **BIOLOGICAL POLLUTANTS:** Mold, dust mites, cockroaches, saliva, or dander from furred animals, pollen. **SMOKE:** Nicotine or wood smoke, candles. **INHALANTS:** Household cleaners, paints, varnishes, perfumes, etc. **EXERCISE:** Although exercise in moderation is beneficial for people with asthma, excessive exercise may trigger an asthma attack—occasionally exercise may produce histamine release, thus triggering an exercise-histamine asthma attack. **EMOTIONAL DISTRESS:** In some people, strong emotion and anxiety can trigger asthma.

*Research shows that the majority of
environmental illnesses such as asthma,
Legionnaire's disease, and humidifier
fever, along with building-related illness
and hypersensitivity pneumonitis are the
direct result of breathing unclean
and polluted air in our homes,
our workplaces, and our schools.*

Where to Look for Biological Pollutants in Your Home

Dust mites, pollen, roaches, molds, and animal dander are everywhere. Chances are great that these biological pollutants are lounging about your home at this very minute. These pollutants may be present:

- In your bedding
- In your pet's bedding
- In and around your air conditioners
- On humidifiers and dehumidifiers
- All over your kitchen
- Up in your attic
- Throughout your laundry room
- Beneath your carpet
- In your basement
- Anywhere that water is leaking
- On your drapes
- On your upholstered furniture.

CHAPTER 2

Dust Mites—Big Diseases Can Come in Small Packages

The Hidden Poop on Dust Mites

Want to hear something truly disgusting? Your house is infested with itsy-bitsy bugs that munch on your skin, burrow into your winter coats, march through your carpets in a microscopic yet relentless army, and even invade the most private sanctuary of all: your bed! Sounds like a nightmare you might have after eating too much spicy food … but dust mites are all too real.

Please understand. I'm not painting this picture to give you nightmares or to ruin your waking hours either. I want you to understand the scope of the enemy so that you'll feel sufficiently motivated to do battle with one of the biggest offenders of air quality in your personal environment.

Dust mites are microscopic organisms that live and breed in warm, moist areas of your home. Having these tiny critters sharing close quarters with you is bad enough, but what's worse is the way they invade and soil your air and make you sick. Actually, it's not the dust mites themselves that cause problems; their feces and cast-off skins are the offending allergens.

Dust mites emit excrement about twenty times a day, and this excrement is so lightweight that it actually floats about in the air. Since there are about 40,000 dust mites per ounce of dust, the amount of dust-mite feces and dead skin that could be permeating the air in your home right now is mind-boggling. What is even more disconcerting is that epidemiological studies indicate that nearly 100 percent of homes and offices are infested with dust mites. That means that every one of us has these little critters in our homes, our offices, and anyplace else where dust tends to settle.

It's not a pleasant thought at all, is it?

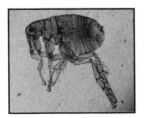

Since there are about 40,000 dust mites per ounce of dust, the amount of dust-mite feces and dead skin that could be permeating the air in your home right now is mind-boggling. Epidemiological studies indicate that nearly 100 percent of homes and offices are infested with dust mites.

The Care and Feeding of These Repugnant Microscopic Critters

Because their name evokes dry, dusty attics that make you choke and cough, you might assume that these tiny beings thrive in arid climates. You'd be wrong. On the contrary, dust mites love humidity, particularly at a level above 50 percent. So those of you living in regions that tend toward humidity—say the tropics or misty climes such as England and the British Isles—are more likely to develop a dust-mite problem than people inhabiting more arid regions, such as desert-dwellers.

The main source of dust-mite food is dander, both human and animal skin flakes. Humans shed approximately one-quarter ounce of dander (dead skin) each week. Interestingly, it has been reported that about 80 percent of the material that you see floating in the air in a shaft of sunlight is actually bits of dead skin. Dust mites are also partial to pollen, fungi, bacteria, moth and butterfly scales, and the skin scales of birds. In laboratories, human, cat, dog, and horse dander have been used as feed to raise dust mites. While they do not drink water in the same way you and I do, they absorb it from the air and the environment. This is why they love humidity; they can eat and drink to their hearts' content. And they do. The higher the relative humidity of their environment, the more sustenance they absorb and the better the chance for their survival.

What this means is that all the places in your home where dead skin collects—bedding, carpets, draperies, and upholstered furniture—may as well be posted with tiny neon signs blinking, "Eat at Joe's!" These areas are actually providing nourishment for the nasty, dangerous, insatiable little creatures. By the way, dust mites have a particular affinity for wool fabrics and rugs. Think about that the next time you snuggle into your favorite oversized wool sweater or curl up on a rug in front of the fire!

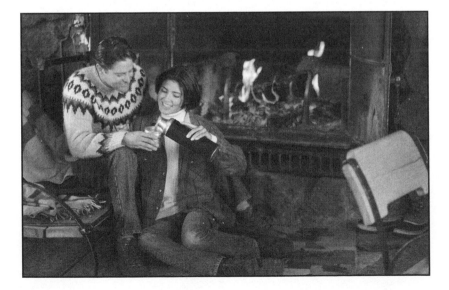

Little Mites Pack a Powerful Health-Risk Punch

Dust mites are so small that their existence wasn't even discovered until 1965. Since then, they have been reported to be the single most causative factor of asthma on a worldwide basis. Epidemiological estimates indicate that dust mites are a causative factor in 50 to 80 percent of asthmatics, as well as in countless cases of eczema, hay fever, and other allergic ailments. Control of dust mites is critical for all allergy-prone people, but it is perhaps most critical for infants. Babies exposed to dust mites in the first year of life may develop a lifelong allergy for which there is no cure, only prevention.

A recent article in the medical journal *Clinical and Experimental Allergy* helps demonstrate a connection between high humidity, which, as previously mentioned, is the ideal environment for dust mites, and the occurrence of asthma. In this study, the authors identified that New Zealand— which has a year-round relative humidity of 82 percent with mild year-round temperatures—has a high prevalence of asthma. Twenty-six percent of adults and 28 percent of thirteen- to fourteen-year-olds reported episodes of wheezing within a twelve-month period. In Wellington, New Zealand, of all of the asthmatics who had a recent hospital admission, 76 percent showed positive skin tests for allergy to the dust mite.

In comparison studies, information from the asthma centers in Great Britain and Scandinavia also revealed higher incidences of dust mite-induced asthma in certain areas of Great Britain where the humidity is higher. It is estimated that in the United Kingdom, one in ten children has asthma and 40 percent of the population will have suffered asthma symptoms at some point before reaching the age of thirty-three.

In another comparison study, measures used to control the dust-mite population in homes—such as whole-house mechanical ventilation with heat-recovery systems and centrifugal force and filtered high-efficiency vacuum cleaners—were implemented in homes in Great Britain and Scandinavia. These measures resulted not only in a significant reduction in the dust-mite population but also in a pronounced clinical reduction in asthma symptoms and a reduced need for medication.

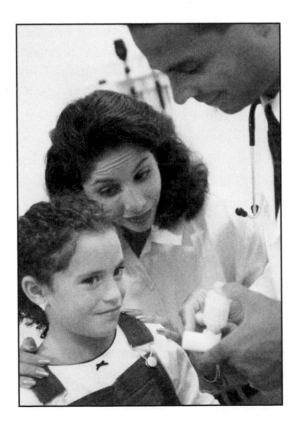

Control of dust mites is most critical for infants. Babies exposed to dust mites in the first year of life may develop a lifelong allergy for which there is no cure, only prevention.

Giving Dust Mites the Boot

This last bit of information—the part about the success our European friends had in reducing the numbers of their unwanted "visitors"—brings us to my favorite part of this chapter: what *you* can do to de-mite-ify *your* home. (Yes, you'll be relieved to hear that there *is* something you can do!)

First, one small caveat: No matter how meticulous a housekeeper you are, *completely* ridding your home and work environment of dust mites is probably not a realistic goal. But you *can* make a big, big dent in their population! Like any unwelcome and intrusive houseguest, the dust mite will only get the hint when you remove its reason for visiting in the first place. Starvation and discomfort are the way to go. The solution is to reduce, to the greatest extent possible, its food supply and its natural habitat. Since it's practically impossible to get rid of *all* dust, a concerted effort to control the mite's breeding habitat can achieve the most favorable results. Think of it as "integrated mite management."

The first step in eradicating your mite infestation may seem counterintuitive. Conventional cleaning, while useful in maintaining the appearance of a tidy home, will not aid your eradication mission. In fact, using a standard vacuum cleaner can actually exacerbate the problem and make allergies worse. That's because standard vacuum cleaners simply stir up the dust, moving the airborne dust mites from one area to another without actually removing them. Plus, the pollutants that escape from the bag when you attempt to empty its contents into the trash will just release more mites into the atmosphere. Caution should be used when removing any bag to prevent more air pollutants. Similarly, standard dusting with a feather duster or cloth only invites more dust, dust mites, and dust-mite waste to take flight through your home, spreading into additional areas and causing a greater likelihood that the offending microscopic particles will be inhaled.

Mite eradication, then, begins with a commitment toward removing unnecessary articles from the home that serve as breeding grounds for the stubborn little allergens. Take inventory of potential mite habitats. You will find that your choices in fabric and filling may have to change. If your home contains lots of the natural fibers that have become so popular in recent years, you may have to switch to synthetic.

For instance, do you use down pillows and wool blankets? While the texture and feel of these products may be inviting, their potential for harboring dust mites is great. Replace them with synthetic fiber products such as those made with nylon or polyester. Natural sheepskin and woolen underlays should also be replaced. You can find comfortable replacements that simulate the natural "comfort properties" of these items in department stores and specialty shops.

If possible, replace all carpeting with wooden, tile, or vinyl flooring. If replacing all your carpet is not feasible—or if you have rugs or other fiber-based floor coverings in your home or office—you should clean the carpet and rugs daily with a high efficiency, high filtration surface cleaner. As mentioned above, using standard vacuum cleaners can actually exacerbate your dust-mite problem because the dust and mites end up being scattered from one area to another.

Most surface cleaners are unlike regular vacuum cleaners which lose airflow and redistribute contaminants.

If you have central air conditioning, keep it running during hot and humid periods. During times of extremely high humidity, such as during the summer months in many regions, it is recommended that a dehumidifier be employed. Your goal is to keep the humidity level below 50 percent.

Pillows, mattresses, and box springs should be covered with an impervious fabric. Acaricide, a product specifically designed to eradicate dust mites, should be applied at least once a month to carpets, mattresses, and upholstered furniture.

Ridding your home of the dust-mite threat is going to take a concerted effort, including some planning, a dedication of time, and most of all, a healthy dose of determination. But if you are willing to follow the steps necessary to control the dust and lower the humidity in your environment, you stand a good chance of relieving yourself, your family, and coworkers of the effects of dust-mite waste allergies. And that's good news for *everyone!*

Nine Steps for Smiting the Mighty Mite

1. Replace all feather and down pillows with synthetic fiber-filled pillows.
2. Replace wool blankets with those made of nylon or cotton cellulose.
3. Cover pillows, mattresses, and box springs with an impervious fabric. These coverings can be bought in any major department store or special allergy store or via allergy product catalogues. Be aware that some allergen covers are more effective than others.
4. At least *once each month,* wash all bedding, including blankets, mattress pads, etc., in hot water (130 degrees Fahrenheit or higher).
5. Change sheets and pillowcases *at least once a week.*
6. Get rid of all carpeting if possible. If this is not feasible, clean the carpet daily with a high efficiency, high filtration surface cleaner. Look for the surface cleaners that are more efficient than HEPA. Remember: *Standard vacuum cleaners generally make allergies worse because they simply move the dust/dust mites airborne from one area to another and "stir in" the dust without actually removing it.* Its important to note most bag cleaners lose air flow when the larger particles clog up the porous openings of the bag thereby reducing air flow. If you can't remove the allergens and toxins then you're not getting the job done.
7. Apply Acaricide (a product that is specific for eradicating dust mites) lightly *at least once per month* to carpets, mattresses, and upholstered

furniture. Acaricides can be bought at most "allergy stores" and are non-allergenic.

8. Use a dehumidifier during high-humidity periods or use central air conditioning. Homes that have the air conditioner on constantly have lower mite counts than non air-conditioned homes. Effective control of mites mandates that the humidity level be below 50 percent.

9. Avoid woolen underlays such as natural sheepskins beneath sheets. These sheepskin underlays, while extremely comfortable, provide a powerful breeding ground for dust mites. New Zealanders, Australians, and people from other "sheep countries" should take particular note of this fact.

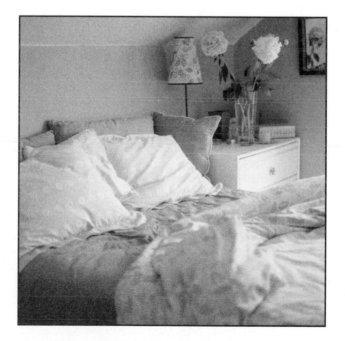

CHAPTER 3

Cockroaches— When Insidious Insects Invade the Indoors

The Creepy Crawlers We Love to Hate

It is the stuff that horror movies are made of—hordes of scurrying cockroaches taking control of your home or apartment, rummaging about on countertops and in kitchen cabinets, crawling out of the fixtures in your bathroom, or, heaven forbid, scampering under the covers of your bed as you sleep. Cockroaches not only spread germs on the surfaces they inhabit, but they also emit airborne allergens that pollute our indoor atmospheres, causing discomfort and disease.

They are the lowliest of the lowly, the creepiest of the creepy, the vilest of the vile. Yes, cockroaches have reached legendary status in our culture. We hate them. We fear them. We use their name as an epithet, aimed at people we truly wish to disparage. And worst of all, we may even feel helpless to control them. Fortunately, we are not truly helpless, just challenged. For the cockroach does, indeed, have several advantages over us.

The Cockroach, a Worthy Opponent

Before we can confront the enemy, we need to understand him. There are some 5,000 species of cockroaches worldwide. They live everywhere in the world. In fact, they can even be found in the North and South Poles, although when the temperature gets extremely cold, they can only survive by taking up residence with human hosts. The pest roaches most commonly found in the West originated in western Asia and northern Africa and spread throughout the world in the luggage of travelers and the cargo holds of wooden vessels.

Roaches come in all sizes and colors. The world's largest roach—a creature I, for one, have no desire to encounter!—is six inches long, has a one-foot wing span, and lives in South America. The smallest roaches are so tiny they often live in ant nests. In the tropics, where many species of roaches live, varieties can be found that are brightly colored red, green, or yellow.

Cockroaches have six legs covered with tiny hairs that give them their sense of touch. They have at least eighteen knees! Many cockroaches have the gift of flight. Their feelers act as noses, allowing them to ferret out food and locate other roaches for amorous encounters.

Cockroaches are fabled to be the only living creature on earth that can survive a nuclear holocaust intact and without missing a beat. And, as with most myths, there actually is something to it. We humans can safely withstand a one-time radiation exposure of up to five rems (a rem is the dosage of radiation that will cause a measurable amount of injury to human tissue). A lethal dose of radiation is 800 rems or more. Cockroach experts report that these adaptable varmints can tolerate a much higher dose. In fact, the lethal dose of radiation for the American cockroach is 67,500 rems, and for the German cockroach, it is between 90,000 and 105,000 rems. So in truth, the amount of radiation that cockroaches can withstand is equivalent to that of a thermonuclear explosion.

Oh, and here's another fascinating, if repulsive, fact: these hearty creatures can even survive for a week after you cut off their heads. It is only their subsequent inability to drink water that deals them the fatal blow. No wonder they don't cower when we chase them around the house with cans of aerosol insecticide!

Roaches are our mortal enemy, and we love to hate them. But the cockroach is far more than merely an unpleasant and annoying reality of urban and even modern suburban life.

Cockroaches and their associated filth pollute our indoor atmosphere and produce dangerous allergens that contribute to asthma and other air-quality-related illnesses.

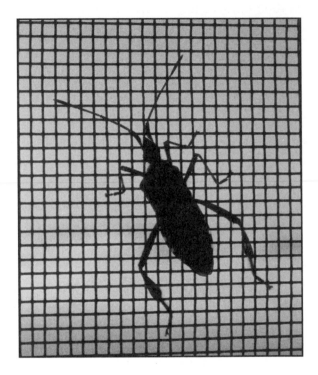

Cockroaches can survive for a week after you cut off their heads. It is only their subsequent inability to drink water that deals them the fatal blow.

Repugnant Roach Disease You Cannot See

We generally think of cockroaches as carriers of disease, pathogenic organisms like bacteria and fungi that can be passed on to humans through surface and food contamination. Salmonella is a common disease carried by cockroaches. However, what may be even more insidious—not to mention harder to control—is the proliferation of cockroach waste and byproducts that travel through the air. Cockroach carcasses and viable roaches in carpeting and rugs cause airborne allergens that pollute our indoor environments, contributing to poor indoor air quality and increased incidence of asthma and other air-quality-related disorders.

If this is news to you, don't feel bad. While cockroach sensitivity has been associated with asthma for more than thirty years, it has been only fairly recently that we have increased our understanding of the extensive dangers posed by cockroach-associated allergens.

Unlike the microscopic dust mite that must be present in large concentrations to wreak its allergenic havoc on our immune systems, asthma symptoms associated with cockroach allergens have a tendency to occur at much lower sensitivity levels. Also, where decreasing the exposure to dust-mite allergens decreases the frequency and severity of asthma episodes, cockroach allergens tend to last for months—even after all signs point to the removal of the pests from the environment. It's all in keeping with the roach's reputation for indefatigability.

And, as if that news weren't bad enough, a recent report by the National Cooperative Inner City Asthma Study noted that removal of cockroach allergen from the home is a most difficult task. In the inner-city areas, re-infestation is a constant problem with new roaches re-entering a seemingly "cockroach-controlled" home from neighboring buildings and apartments.

Furthermore, high levels of cockroach allergens can easily be sent airborne with minimal disturbance. Even the act of running a conventional vacuum cleaner can send the offending particles flying. The miniscule particles—averaging ten microns in diameter—are simply too small to be contained by conventional cleaning techniques. Only a high efficiency, high filtration cleaner is capable of controlling the airborne allergens of this size. Standard cleaning and vacuuming, while reducing the number of roaches visible to the eye, can actually release more of the microscopic allergens into the atmosphere than would have been there had you not cleaned, dusted, or vacuumed at all.

Does that mean there is nothing that can be done? Certainly not. But the problem is so pervasive—particularly in low-income, multi-family housing complexes—that the concerted and well-coordinated efforts of landlords, public-health officials, and residents is needed to even begin to approach a systemic solution to what is more and more often a life-threatening problem. In general, studies show that in order to reduce asthma morbidity, cockroach allergen must be reduced by at least tenfold, and these reductions must be sustained for six months or more. It is only through the coordinated efforts of all concerned that cockroach-induced airborne morbidity can be reduced.

The Public Health System's Role in Roach Eradication

In the inner cities, cockroach infestation is an insidious public-health matter. For any headway to be made in the control of the problem, city, state, and federal government health agencies and health-insurance companies need to come together to launch an all-out attack on biological indoor pollutants, particularly pollutants caused by cockroaches. Public health must take a stand against indoor air pollution in order to protect our citizenry. I encourage citizens to form neighborhood air-pollution watches much along the same vein as the crime-watch groups that have sprung up all over the country. Start petition drives and write, call, and email your state and federal legislators, as well as your local elected officials. Raise their awareness of these important health issues.

Readying Your Home to Reject Roaches

Now that you've learned how creepy cockroaches really are—as if you needed to be convinced!—you're probably wondering how you can get rid of these formidable foes. In fact, since you now know a lot more about their resilient nature, you may be wondering if eradication is even possible. You'll be happy to hear that you can, indeed, root out roaches. It'll just take some determination and vigilance.

There are several affirmative steps that the house- or apartment-dweller can take to make cockroaches feel less comfortable in his or her home. While removing the roaches won't immediately rid your home of the allergens, at least it will serve to decrease the amount of new material entering the atmosphere. The best course of action to take is following a plan that includes eradication of roaches that occurs in combination with air filtration.

Dry Them Out

The first line of defense is a good offense, and the easiest way to offend a cockroach is to take away its water supply. As mentioned previously, the resilient creatures can live without a head, but they can't live without a drink of water. So the first logical step to take in your fight against cockroach infestation is to dry them out. Pick up pet water dishes at night, the time when cockroaches are most likely to come out of their hiding places looking for a drink. Fix leaky faucets and pipes and thoroughly inspect your home for any other water-retaining or water-producing appliances. Does water collect under the kitchen or bathroom sinks? Under the refrigerator? Are there any puddles present by the washing machine or dishwasher? Remember, just a little water can quench a cockroach's thirst, allowing it to survive and even to propagate for up to seven days, even if its food supply is taken away.

Starve Them Out

Next, you can try to starve them out. Take care not to leave food out overnight. All food should be either refrigerated or placed in tightly sealed containers. Clean kitchen counters and sinks with soapy water and restrict food consumption to one or two areas of the house, such as the kitchen or dining room. Eating and drinking in the living room and bedrooms just increases the likelihood that crumbs or water will inadvertently be left out for these most hearty of unwelcome pests.

Evict Them

Serve eviction notices to the cockroaches harboring in your home. Get rid of paper and cardboard items such as newspapers, grocery bags, and boxes where roaches love to hide. Remove or repair loose wallpaper, a typical hiding place and breeding ground for cockroaches, particularly in older homes and apartments. Seal cracks and spaces in walls around electrical outlets, windowsills, and baseboards. If you've seen cockroaches in toasters or toaster ovens, send them a chilly goodbye by wrapping the appliance in a plastic bag and storing it in the freezer. This is also a good idea for any small box or electrical item, such as a clock, radio, or small television set. In the wintertime, you can even seal up these items in a plastic garbage bag and put them outside.

Clear the Air of Them

Invest in a high efficiency, high filtration portable room air cleaner. This will rid the atmosphere of the remnants of the microscopic cockroach allergens that are making you sick. Apply non-allergic toxic pesticides on a regular basis and distribute cockroach traps throughout the house.

See? You *can* get these hateful household pests out of your life. It takes a bit of work, and sure, the neighbors may wonder why your microwave is sitting on the front porch in the middle of January—but who cares? Knowing that you and your family are enjoying a roach-free existence is worth it!

The Resilient Roach: Some Skin-Crawling Factoids

It's true: cockroaches can survive a nuclear holocaust. The lethal dose of radiation for the American cockroach is 67,500 rems, and for the German cockroach, it is between 90,000 and 105,000 rems. Compare that to 800 rems for human beings.

Cockroaches can survive for a week after you cut off their heads. It is only their subsequent inability to drink water that deals them the fatal blow.

Cockroach allergens tend to last for months, even after all signs point to the removal of the pests from the environment.

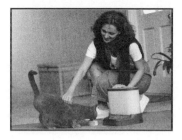

Nine Steps to Reduce Raunchy Roach Allergens

1. Eliminate the cockroach's water supply. Empty pet water dishes at night, seal all pipes, and fix any leaky appliances.
2. Secure all food products in the refrigerator and in tightly sealed containers.
3. Restrict food consumption to select areas in your home and clean up thoroughly after each meal. Avoid eating at your office and workstation.
4. Remove cardboard boxes, newspapers, and paper grocery bags from your home.
5. Seal cracks and spaces in walls around electrical outlets, window sills, and baseboards.
6. Remove or repair loose wallpaper.
7. Wrap small appliances that may harbor roaches in plastic and store them in the freezer when not in use.
8. Apply Abamectin—a non-allergenic, non-toxic pesticide—to all cockroach-infested areas on a *monthly* basis.
9. Invest in a high efficiency, high filtration portable room air cleaner. Remember: Airborne allergens produced by cockroaches are often present for several months after all visible evidence of roach infestation is gone.

CHAPTER 4

Molds— Unsettling Spores that Soil the Air

The Mold Menace

Wherever you are at this very moment—sitting in your living room, relaxing in your bedroom, browsing in a bookstore, or sipping a nice hot cup of joe in your favorite coffee shop—you are breathing in microscopic mold spores. I am almost certain of it.

Mold is a common fungus and can be found just about anywhere. In fact, mold has always been with us and probably always will be. Mold, it seems, has been a major cause of a whole slew of maladies since the beginning of time. If you don't believe me, just turn to your Bible (see Leviticus, Chapters 11–14) for perhaps the first recorded attempts to control mold infestation.

We usually think of mold as the unsightly and smelly green fuzz that forms on week-old bread and on those forgotten chunks of cheese that somehow got squirreled away in the back of the refrigerator. Maybe when you think of mold, you think of that creeping green/black slime that is readily visible on roof tiles and bathroom walls, perhaps in an area where you've had a leak of some kind. But, in reality, mold is all of this … and much, much more. It is among the most widespread of living organisms and is prevalent all over your home, workplace, and children's school. Mold is a hearty allergen that can grow on virtually any substance anywhere at any time. If you've got moisture, then you've got mold. And if you've got mold, chances are good that you're breathing in mold spores at this very moment.

While some molds are visible to the naked eye and even emit that acrid, musty, mildew scent—the kind that makes you want to cover your nose and mouth and flee from the room—not all molds are so easy to detect. In fact, mold is often a hidden menace—sneaking up on you and infiltrating your environment and your air, causing discomfort and disease. Indoor mold is present year-round, and since airborne mold spores are invisible to the naked eye and have no discernible odor, these tiny particles can wreak havoc on your respiratory system and even on your immune system without you ever realizing that they are there.

Mold can be a hidden menace— sneaking up on you and infiltrating your environment and your air, causing discomfort and disease. ... These tiny particles can wreak havoc on your respiratory system and even on your immune system without you ever realizing that they are there.

Molds' Hunger for Humidity

Molds thrive in dark, warm, humid areas. They can be found in the shower, on bathroom walls, and even inside your mattress! Molds live and grow on air conditioners and humidifiers, in areas beneath sinks, in refrigerator drain pans, inside garbage cans, behind baseboards and walls, and even beneath concrete. If you keep kitty litter in your house, chances are there is some mold in there as well. The same holds true for birdcages and other environments where moisture, in combination with shedding or molting household creatures, produces a common recipe for mold reproduction. Slacking off on housekeeping also can create an inviting environment for mold to grow. Leaving dishes stacked in the sink or allowing food to fester in the open invites mold to make a home in your kitchen. Forgetting to take out the trash on a daily basis or keeping a trash compactor full can increase the likelihood that this fungus will appear.

Mold may also be present in other areas of your home. Look closely at your window treatments. Even if you don't see or smell anything "funny," mold could be doing its dirty deeds on your draperies. Ever walk into an attic or open the closet doors and get that musty airless sensation? It's probably due to the existence of mold in these poorly ventilated environments. Thinking of enjoying a soak in the hot tub? Or finally planning to spend the afternoon catching up on all that laundry? It's likely that you'll be sharing your relaxing soak or spending your laundry day in the unwelcome company of mold.

And your efforts to reduce your air-conditioning bills by installing ceiling fans and turning up the thermostat may be saving you money, but have you noticed that your sinuses have been bothering you more? Or your headaches have returned? It's likely that your frugality has created the perfect environment for mold to reproduce. Since moisture-loving molds can feed on any organic matter, all you need to provide a perfect home for this most menacing miscreant is an environment where the humidity exceeds 40 percent, where there is plenty of organic matter for its nourishment, and where there is poor ventilation. Think about the places where you work, study, and sleep and chances are these environments are perfect for the production of mold.

Moisture-loving molds can feed on any organic matter. All you need to provide a perfect home for this most menacing miscreant is an environment where the humidity exceeds 40 percent, where there is plenty of organic matter for its nourishment, and where there is poor ventilation.

Maladies Caused by the Malevolent Mold

Molds reproduce by releasing their tiny spores into the air. The spores settle on organic matter and proceed to grow into new mold clusters. A single germinating mold can produce hundreds of thousands of airborne spores, sometimes in less than a week. Perpetual inhalation of mold spores in closed environments such as homes, workplaces, and schools can lead to chronic sinusitis, as well as a host of respiratory diseases, including asthma. In fact, since many molds are present at the same time of year as pollen, people often mistake their sneezing and wheezing for hay fever when in fact these symptoms are caused by the malevolent mold. People with chronic, recurrent sinusitis should ask their doctors to culture their sinuses for fungi (molds). Until recently, the prevailing medical opinion was that only 6 to 7 percent of all chronic sinusitis was attributed to molds. That theory has now been discounted. A recent study conducted at the Mayo Clinic found that a full 93 percent of patients with chronic sinusitis had allergic *fungal* sinusitis. It turns out that it was the *mold* that was causing the problem after all!

Inhaling mold can affect more than just your sinuses. Have you ever felt tired and irritable for no apparent reason? Do you ever get rashes and not know where they come from? Do you suffer from more headaches than usual? If the answer to any of these questions is yes, then it is worth your while to determine whether the existence of mold in your indoor environment could be the cause. Chronic fatigue syndrome and certain autoimmune disorders have been attributed to mold exposure. Mold can make you break out in a rash and can even cause or exacerbate existing skin conditions such as eczema. The presence of mold could furnish the explanation for your headaches and that hard-to-describe general lethargy you've been experiencing.

As if these symptoms and maladies aren't bad enough, some types of molds can even be deadly! For example, if stachybotrys mold spores are inhaled into the lungs, they can weaken the blood vessels and cause bleeding in the lungs. This type of mold is wet, black, and slimy—the kind that smears when you touch it. Exposure can be fatal for infants and pregnant women. Symptoms such as coughing up blood

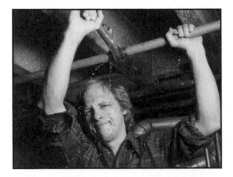

and nosebleeds can be signs of stachybotrys poisoning. This deadly mold is often found on leaky pipes or on the walls or ceiling where high levels of moisture can be found.

Since many molds are present at the same time of year as pollen, people often mistake their sneezing and wheezing for hay fever when in fact these symptoms are caused by the malevolent mold.

Poor Ventilation Is a Mold's Best Friend

Nowhere is the existence of mold more menacing than in our schools where scores of children are exposed to these sickness-causing spores every single day. The Environmental Protection Agency (EPA) has identified mold exposure as precariously prevalent in our nation's schools, accounting in part for the rising rates of asthma and chronic sinusitis in schoolchildren, teachers, and other school employees. In fact, in 1995 the EPA randomly surveyed schools across the nation and estimated that *half* of all of our schools are polluted! This mold-induced indoor air pollution that is now found in our schools likely began with the energy crisis in the seventies. At that time, in a well-meaning attempt to reduce energy use, many schools began to reduce indoor airflow. In addition, and probably as a result of budgetary constraints, air filters on school heating and air-conditioning systems units are not being changed on a regular basis. This reduction in airflow, coupled with the failure to properly maintain air-filtration maintenance systems, ends up aggravating air-quality problems and causing more problems than they were supposed to solve. As

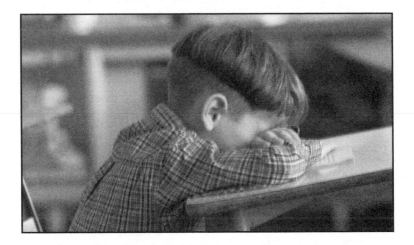

it turns out, these unhealthy practices are creating an unsafe environment in our schools where mold is making a comeback and sickness is following suit.

Poor ventilation is not just a problem in our schools. Take a moment to examine your own home and office heating and air-conditioning ducts. Do you detect a musty odor? Is there any indication that moisture is present in or around the ducts or the unit? Think about it—do you remember the last time you changed the air filters? If these filters become wet, mold and mildew can begin sprouting within three hours, spewing mold spores everywhere the ventilation system reaches!

I cannot emphasize this point enough: The heating and air-conditioning ducts in our schools, homes, and workplaces *must* be inspected on a regular basis to insure that they are free from molds and other pollutants. Mold pollution of our indoor air is greatly under-recognized as a major health hazard! And prevention through vigilance must be employed if we are to keep our indoor environments safe and free of disease-causing mold spores.

The Environmental Protection Agency has identified mold exposure as precariously prevalent in our nation's schools, accounting in part for the rising rates of asthma and chronic sinusitis in schoolchildren, teachers, and other school employees.

Giving Mold the Old Heave-Ho

Just because it seems that unwanted mold has been around forever, and was even causing discomfort during the days when David was slaying Goliath, doesn't mean that you have to continue to let it disrupt your life and make you and your loved ones ill. To accomplish some of the tasks I am recommending, you may have to become a modern-day David and take on the Goliath of your local school board, apartment building superintendent, or office management staff. But this chapter should arm you with all the ammunition you need to convince the people in charge of your indoor environments that an ounce of ventilation maintenance can be worth a pound of benefits. A mold-free indoor environment will result in a reduction in sick leave and school absences, making up for the savings supposedly realized by reduced energy usage or less stringent maintenance of ventilation systems. You can take on many of the steps I am going to mention on your own, especially if you own your home. And for those requiring the complicity of others, don't be afraid to take a stand. Remember: there is no greater crusade than the crusade to safeguard your health and the health of your family and coworkers.

One fairly simple step you can take to control mold is to reduce the humidity level in your home or workplace by the use of a dehumidifier. Care should be taken to reduce the humidity level to below 50 percent. Increasing your air-conditioning use is also helpful. Remember: while it may seem like raising the thermostat is a good cost-conscious way of reducing your utility bills, what you may end up doing is increasing the chances that mold spores will be present to

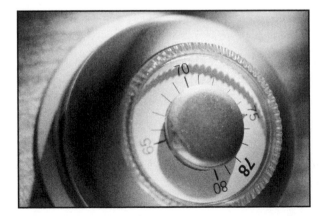

make you sick. That seems like an awfully high price to pay for a little reduction in your utility payments.

It is also useful to add electrostatic air filters to central heating and air-conditioning systems, but be certain to choose a system that does not produce ozone. This will prevent the re-circulation of mold spores throughout the enclosed environment. And while we are talking about control of mold spores through ventilation-system maintenance, remember that routine cleaning and changing air filters can do a lot to make your environment mold resistant. As an added safeguard, it is recommended that a portable high efficiency, high filtration air cleaner be utilized to clear airborne mold spores from your indoor environments.

Clean potential moisture-trapping and mold-growing sites with a solution of one part bleach and four parts water. Areas that should be cleaned with this solution include refrigerator drain pans, bathtubs and hot tubs, areas around washing machines and dishwashers, under sinks, and around any surfaces where water tends to collect. If you cannot get rid of all standing water in your home, you may even want to add a bit of bleach or mold inhibitor to areas where water is certain to collect—such as air-conditioning ducts or drip pans.

Inspect your carpet, ceiling tiles, and draperies. Where mold is present, consider replacing the offending items or using a bleach solution to thoroughly kill off any mold or fungus that is present.

You are in more control of your indoor environment than you may think. And when you think of the myriad diseases and maladies that can result from inhaling mold spores, there seems to be little choice other than to take a stand, load your slingshot, and, like a spore-eradicating David, slay the mold that is polluting your air.

Mold-Causing Maladies

Do you or your family members experience any of these symptoms? If so, mold may be the menace that is making you sick.

- Chronic recurrent sinusitis
- Wheezing, sneezing, or other "hay fever" symptoms
- Unexplained irritability and/or fatigue
- Headaches with no apparent cause or explanation
- Unexplained rashes or other skin conditions such as eczema
- Chronic fatigue syndrome
- Asthma

Think about it—do you remember the last time you changed your air filters? If these filters become wet, mold and mildew can begin sprouting within three hours, spewing mold spores everywhere the ventilation system reaches.

Ten Steps to Slaying the Menacing Mold Spore

1. Clean all areas where mold might grow—anywhere water collects or moisture is high—with a bleach or mold-inhibitor solution. Make sure you remove all visible mold stains. If using bleach, it should be diluted: one part bleach to four parts water.

2. Employ a dehumidifier to reduce the level of humidity in your indoor environment to below 50 percent.

3. Replace all water-stained ceiling tiles.

4. Check beneath carpet for trapped moisture. If the carpet is retaining water, replace it with fresh carpet and remove the source of the water.

5. Do not let water stand in air-conditioning ducts or refrigerator drip pans. Where water remains, add bleach or a mold inhibitor to the water.

6. Use a portable, high efficiency, high filtration air cleaner to clear out airborne mold spores.

7. Consider adding an electrostatic air filter to your central heating and air-conditioning systems to prevent re-circulation of mold spores.

8. Remove all sources of moisture from homes or workplaces.

9. Keep thermostats low enough to ensure that air is circulating. Reduce your reliance on ceiling fans and let the air conditioning run as much as possible.

10. If you need to, fight city hall. Appeal to your school board and other government agencies to keep your school ventilation systems in clean and good working order. Educate your office manager and building superintendent about the dangers of mold spores. If they are resistant, give them a copy of this book!

CHAPTER 5

Pollen—When Outdoor Allergens Poison Indoor Air

'Tis the Season ... for Sneezing

Ah, don't you just love springtime? After a long dark winter of short days and frigid nights, after shoveling mounds of snow and traversing perilous icy roadways, after bundling up layer upon layer of insulated clothing topped off with a coat, hat, and scarf every time you venture out-of-doors, it is finally spring ... the much anticipated and welcomed time when life renews itself. The birds are chirping and the flowers are blooming ... and if you're like thousands of people with pollen allergies, you are utterly miserable because you are sneezing and wheezing and hacking up a storm.

Maybe you look forward to the lazy days of summer ... loading up the family in the SUV (in my day, it was a wood-paneled five-door station wagon supreme) and heading off to the Grand Canyon or the Great Smoky Mountains or even to Disney World for a day or two with the world-famous mouse and some of his whimsical cartoon friends. But if you suffer from summer-season allergies, it's likely that sinus discomfort will interfere with your summer frolics, turning an otherwise joyful time into a season fraught with nasal nuisance.

If you are like me, it is the autumn that you most look forward to. After a long, hot summer when the sweltering heat and air-so-thick-you-could-cut-a-knife-through-it humidity makes even the simplest tasks daunting, it is finally getting cool and crisp enough to enjoy the outdoors once again. Autumn is a time when nature explodes into magnificent glorious color schemes. The landscape bursts brilliantly into almost magical arrangements of orange and yellow leaves. But if you are an allergy sufferer, you'll be forced to wonder at the marvels of the fall foliage from a safe distance, loathe to enjoy the outdoors when the result is certain to be pollen-induced misery.

Each spring, summer, and fall, thousands of people experience the runny nose, watery eyes, and attacks of sneezing associated with an allergy to pollen. Unfortunately, you do not have much control over the proliferation of pollen in the outdoor environment. As you will see, even if you succeed in creating a foliage-free sanctuary for yourself in your own backyard or immediate outdoor environment, that pesky pollen, due to its propensity to travel great distances by hitching a ride on the wind, will nevertheless probably find you. But you can do a lot to keep your indoor areas pollen free and at least create a safe haven from the dastardly little pollen demons. Before we explore the steps to prevent an indoor pollen invasion, it is useful to know something about this allergy-causing adversary.

Even if you succeed in creating a foliage-free sanctuary for yourself in your own backyard or immediate outdoor environment, that pesky pollen, due to its propensity to travel great distances by hitching a ride on the wind, will nevertheless probably find you.

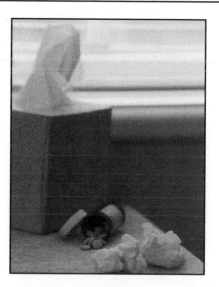

Pernicious Pollen and Its Annoying Attributes

Where does pollen come from? What exactly is it, and how can something so small make you feel so bad?

To understand how pollen is produced and why it affects so many of us in such negative ways, we need to explore the amorous habits of some common varieties of vegetation. Many of these plants, grasses, and trees release tiny reproductive structures into the air in the spring, summer, and fall. These structures contain the male gamete (male DNA) that, upon landing on the female portion of the plant, grass, or tree, completes the fertilization necessary for reproduction. These reproductive structures are known as pollen grains. Though they are microscopic in size—varying from fifteen to 100 micros each—they form a pollen powder, the tiniest portion of which can pack a disproportionately powerful punch. Pollen powder can contain thousands of these pollen grains. In fact, it has been reported that a single ragweed plant—one of the biggest sources of seasonal allergies—can generate as many as a million pollen grains a day! To make matters even worse, these tiny grains like to travel. In fact, they've been known to travel for many hundreds of miles. Samples of ragweed pollen have been detected two miles high in the air and as far as 400 miles out at sea. And that's why your attempts to rid your yard and its surroundings of pollen-producing plants won't necessarily mean you succeed in reducing your outdoor exposure.

You have probably heard your local weatherman or seen an article in your local newspaper refer to the pollen count.

Pollen counts are obtained through the use of air-sampling equipment that captures airborne pollens. The number of pollen grains collected are then counted, logged, and reported to your local media. Reporting the pollen count is an art as much as it is a science, and the results reported in your area can vary depending on the time of day the count is taken (concentrations are usually highest in the morning), the strength of the wind at the time of testing, and weather conditions such as temperature, precipitation, and humidity. When the pollen count is high, people with pollen sensitivities are often quite miserable. Typical symptoms include itching, burning eyes, a continuous runny nose (allergic rhinitis), and paroxysms of sneezing with as many as twenty-five to thirty sneezes during a single episode.

The National Allergy Bureau updates its pollen-count data three times a week. For information about the current count in your area, you can contact the Bureau by calling 1-800-976-5536 or by checking pollen counts on Internet sites such as www.weather.com.

Pollen has been known to travel for many hundreds of miles. Samples of ragweed pollen have been detected two miles high in the air and as far as 400 miles out at sea.

Why Hay Fever? It's Not from Hay, and It Doesn't Cause a Fever

Seasonal allergic rhinitis is often referred to as "hay fever," "rose fever," or "pollen fever." Dr. John Bostock, a British physician, coined the term "hay fever" in the nineteenth century. And although this term is still widely used, it is a bit of a misnomer. According to some sources, Dr. Bostock first noticed that the allergy symptoms seemed to occur right around haying season and that these symptoms were similar to those associated with a cold. And even though it was grass pollen, not the hay, that caused the patients' symptoms, and even though the cold-like symptoms were not accompanied by a fever, the term "hay fever" became accepted shorthand. References to "rose fever" and "pollen fever" followed suit, but all refer to what we now know to be allergic rhinitis.

Weeds are the greatest producers of allergenic pollen in North America. While ragweed is the most prolific pollen-producing weed, sagebrush, redroot pigweed, lamb's quarters, tumbleweed, and English plantain are also offenders. Some grasses are also high pollen-producers. While nearly 1,000 species of grass grow in North America, just a handful is actually responsible for seasonal allergies. These include Kentucky bluegrass, Johnson grass, Bermuda grass, orchard grass, timothy grass, redtop grass, and sweet vernal grass. Pollen-producing trees to watch out for include oak, ash, elm, hickory, pecan, box elder, and mountain cedar.

Hay Fever—Sounding the (False) Alarm

id you know that, in a strange sort of way, your body's reaction to pollen is its way of protecting you? Sounds strange, I know. It's hard to believe that your itchy eyes, runny nose, sneezing, hacking cough, and accompanying headaches are actually reactions by your immune system to a perceived threat to your health and well-being.

When an allergic person inhales pollen (or other allergens, such as mold spores, for that matter), the immune system thinks these foreign bodies are somehow threatening your survival. Like a soldier armed and ready for battle, the immune system comes to full attention and gets ready for an onslaught of further attacks by producing antibodies. Your immune system has a whole arsenal to protect you from a slew of perceived threats and may produce an antibody specific to each offending allergy-producing substance such as ragweed or tumbleweed. The antibody tells your system to fight the offending agent with a variety of chemicals, including histamine. Within minutes you end up with a stuffy nose followed by the sniffles. Over the next several hours, you may find yourself having what we commonly refer to as a full-fledged allergy attack when in reality the symptoms are caused by your body's reaction to a perceived attack already in progress. Ironic, isn't it?

Seek a Specialist to Reduce Symptoms

There is a lot of information out there to assist pollen-allergy patients with controlling symptoms. Unless you live in an igloo at the Arctic Circle or confine yourself to some sort of allergy-free bubble, the chances are slim that you are going to be able to rid your environment completely of pollen and other allergens. Shipping yourself out to sea won't work because, as was pointed out earlier, ragweed spores have been located many miles offshore. While I will be giving you some suggestions for ridding your indoor sanctuary of this pesky allergen, if allergies make you so miserable so as to interfere with the quality of your life, you should sit down with an allergy specialist to develop a comprehensive treatment plan. The allergist will likely conduct a series of tests to pinpoint, to the greatest extent possible, the triggers for your allergy symptoms. While most allergy symptoms can be controlled by medications—such as antihistamines and decongestants or nasal steroid sprays—properly prescribed by a competent allergy physician, in severe cases, your allergist may recommend allergy immunotherapy, after discussing a plan for allergy avoidance. Allergy immunotherapy usually consists of a series of desensitizing injections over a protracted period of time. While nobody looks forward to having a needle stuck in his or her arm once or twice a week, undergoing these desensitizing injections can provide a world of relief for individuals for whom other therapies have proven ineffective.

Nobody looks forward to having a needle stuck in his or her arm once or twice a week, but undergoing these desensitizing injections can provide a world of relief for individuals for whom other therapies have proven ineffective.

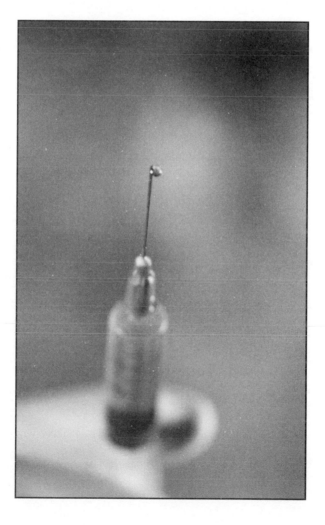

Keeping Pollen in Its Place

If you must spend time outdoors during the height of pollen season, you should schedule your time outside so that you encounter as little exposure to these allergens as possible. Monitor the pollen-count reports for your area and avoid being out-of-doors when the concentration is particularly high. Because wind can stir pollen around and increase your chances of exposure, wear a mask over your nose and mouth on windy days. A mask should also be worn when doing any type of yard work—such as mowing the lawn or raking leaves. Look for a mask that will protect you from particles as small as ten or twelve microns and be sure to clean or change the mask regularly.

Your home should be your pollen-free sanctuary. However, it will be necessary to make a concerted effort to control your indoor environment if you are to experience relief from the perils that persist outside during the time your seasonal allergies are most severe. First, make a habit of removing your shoes and clothing immediately upon arriving at your home. Taking a shower when you get home will also remove any lingering pollen that has adhered to your skin and hair.

Hair actually acts as a magnet for pollen, so thoroughly washing your hair, especially before bedtime, should serve to protect you from spreading microscopic pollen spores to your bedsheets and pillows. You may also want to try putting a leave-in conditioner on your hair before you venture outside. This added protective coating will make it more difficult for pollen to attach to your hair in the first place.

Dry your clothes and linens in the dryer rather than leaving them outside on a clothesline. While the clean fresh

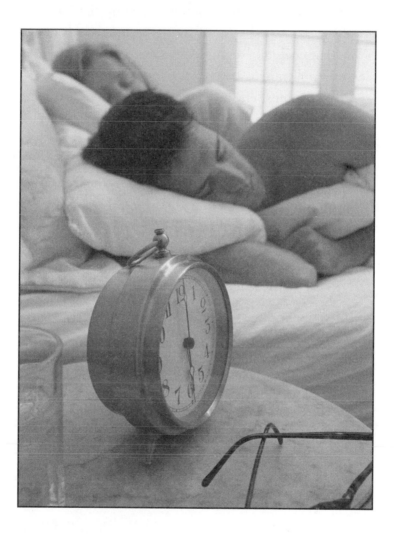

scent of air-drying can be pleasant at first, what's the point of fresh-smelling sheets when you're so congested that you can't really smell anything anyway?

Windows should be kept closed during pollen season, and you should keep the air conditioning running as much as possible. There is a temptation to "open up the house," especially at those first signs of spring, or to take advantage of those first cool fall evenings, but keep in mind that you'll be inviting pollen in as well.

One of the most effective and efficient ways for dealing with pollen sensitivity is to invest in a portable, high efficiency, high filtration air cleaner. A high-quality air cleaner is especially recommended for use in your bedroom. If you suffer from pollen allergies, you know that allergy attacks can rob you of a good night's sleep, thereby magnifying the intensity of your allergic symptoms. By clearing the air in your home and removing lingering pollen particles, you will be assuring yourself of a safe allergy-free sanctuary throughout the dreaded pollen season.

There is a temptation to "open up the house," especially at those first signs of spring, or to take advantage of those first cool fall evenings, but keep in mind that you'll be inviting pollen in as well.

Seven Steps to Protect Your Premises from Pollen

1. Monitor your area's pollen count and reduce outdoor activities when concentrations are high, and reduce indoor pollen counts with a surface cleaner.

2. Cover your mouth and nose with a mask on windy days or when working outside. The mask should protect you from particles as small as fifteen microns.

3. Remove shoes and clothing as soon as you enter your home. Immediately take a shower to avoid spreading pollen once you are indoors.

4. Because hair is a pollen magnet, wash hair regularly and coat hair with a leave-in conditioner to repel pollen.

5. Dry your clothes and linens in the clothes dryer rather than using an outdoor clothesline.

6. Always keep windows closed during pollen season. Resist the temptation to "air out the house."

7. Use a portable, high efficiency, high filtration air cleaner to rid your home of any pollen that may make its way indoors.

CHAPTER 6

Animal Allergens—The Perils of Keeping Indoor Pets

The Sensitive Subject of Pet-Produced Allergens

I know that I am treading on sensitive ground when it comes to discussing how to prevent pet allergens from polluting your indoor environment. If you, or a member of your family, suffers from allergic reactions brought on by certain pets, the solution—or at least part of the solution—has to include a rethinking of your pets' habitat, especially if his habitat is also your home.

Maybe you have a favorite furry friend who lounges with you on the Lazy Boy or sleeps at the foot of your bed. I have an acquaintance who would rather cuddle up to her cocker spaniel, I think, than snuggle up to her spouse. And I know a widower whose favorite cat has been his faithful companion ever since the loss of his dear wife may years ago. The sweet Siamese greets him at the door when he gets home from work and provides a purring reminder that he is not alone as they spend their evenings together in front of the television. While it cannot be denied that pets can play important roles in our lives, I would be remiss if I did not point out the potential problems caused by maintaining such close relationships with these furry friends.

In Western culture, it has become increasingly popular to share living space with pets. Dogs, cats, rodents, and rabbits—you name it! If there is a furry animal that comes even close to approximating something warm and cute,

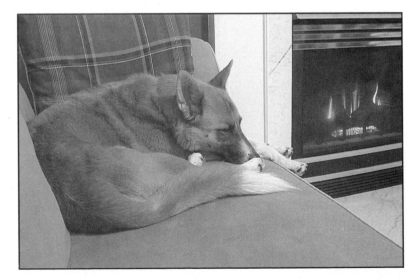

somebody has one, and it probably is living in his or her home. Unfortunately, furred animals (especially cats) can cause as much allergic sensitization and disease in the home environment as the easy-to-disdain dust mites, cockroaches, and molds that were previously discussed in this book. It's true that we don't give our roaches and dust mites names, and mold doesn't welcome us at the door after a long day's work or offer us unconditional love and acceptance, whether we deserve it or not. So don't think for a minute that I am going to try to convince all you pet lovers out there that Rover should be treated in the same vein as a cockroach or dust mite, even though the symptoms and diseases resulting from pet-produced allergens may be just as severe.

Studies show that as many as 15 percent of us have allergies to cats or dogs. A recent survey conducted in the United States revealed that about two million of us are allergic to cats but choose to have one live in our homes anyway. And when we are informed that our severe allergy symptoms are caused by our pets, four out of five of us keep living with our pets nevertheless, and we will likely even get *another* similar pet after the previous pet dies. It may take a life-threatening bout of asthma or some other kind of wake-up call before the person affected by pet allergen undertakes the necessary steps to protect his or her health.

Furred animals (especially cats), can cause as much allergic sensitization and disease in the home environment as the easy-to-disdain dust mites, cockroaches, and molds.

Fur Is Not the Offending Foe

If you or someone in your family is suffering from an allergic pet sensitivity, you owe it to yourself to explore what you can do to reduce, if not eliminate, the cause. Of course, you must understand what in the world is causing your allergic symptoms in the first place. Here's a bit of news that might come as a surprise—it's not the fur that you're allergic to at all! In fact, contrary to popular notion, there is no such thing as a "hypo-allergenic" animal. "Big-haired" animals such as Persian cats or shedding dogs don't make you more allergic than, say, a short-haired pointer or one of those furless wrinkle-skinned cats. (Remember the funny-looking feline in that Austin Powers movie?)

That's because what causes all the sneezing and the wheezing is actually a protein contained in the animal's skin and, believe it or not, its saliva and urine. The more the animal licks its fur, a common self-grooming behavior undertaken by many animals and especially by cats, the more saliva-laden protein and concomitant allergens are released.

A recent survey conducted in the United States revealed that about two million of us are allergic to cats but choose to have one live in our homes anyway.

Urine is the major source of allergies caused by guinea pigs, gerbils, mice, and rats, which many people keep as pets. When the substance carrying the protein—saliva, urine, or skin dander—dries, the proteins float into the air and become a source of indoor air pollution.

As we saw in previous chapters, the dust-mite population in homes with pets increases due to the fact that pet dander is a favorite dust-mite food. Animals can also bring pollen into the home on their fur and paws, adding to your pollen pollution problem.

Because allergies to animals can take as long as two years to develop, we often exhibit pet-allergy symptoms but, understandably, do not attribute them to the pet. Also, it has been shown that pet allergens can remain in carpets and furniture for up to six weeks following the pet's removal from the premises. The result can be that previous pet owners who are continuing to suffer from their allergy symptoms end up wondering if their pet allergy was just a figment of their imagination.

What causes all the sneezing and the wheezing is actually a protein contained in the animal's skin and, believe it or not, its saliva and urine. The more the animal licks its fur, a common self-grooming behavior undertaken by many animals and especially by cats, the more saliva-laden protein and concomitant allergens are released.

Even the Petless Can Be Prone to Animal Allergies

People who do not count themselves among the growing number of indoor pet owners may still feel the effects of others' animal cohabitation. Pet-keeping individuals regularly bring pet allergens into pet-free environments, such as day-care centers and schools, where pets are not allowed. The pet allergens attach to the pet owners' clothing and other personal items and contaminate these pet-free zones, causing allergic reactions in people who have sought out these environments for the precise reason of avoiding this type of contamination. It is believed that this residual effect of keeping pets indoors is responsible for undetected pet-allergy reactions in individuals who have made the conscious choice to avoid pet-allergen exposure.

In some countries, the pet-allergic are provided with safe havens from these allergens. For example, in Sweden preschool children that are allergic to furred pets, as well as other allergens, are placed in special "allergen-avoidance" day-care centers. In these centers, neither children nor staff members are allowed to have furred pets in their homes. The general cleaning practices are more extensive than in conventional day-care centers, and even carpets are forbidden. High efficiency, high filtration air cleaners are typically used to further reduce the presence of all allergens, including those produced by furred animals. While these practices may seem a bit "over the top" to American pet-loving sensibilities, the result has been a healthier environment for the children, fewer cases of asthma, less need for asthma medication, and a reduction in absenteeism due to allergy-causing illness.

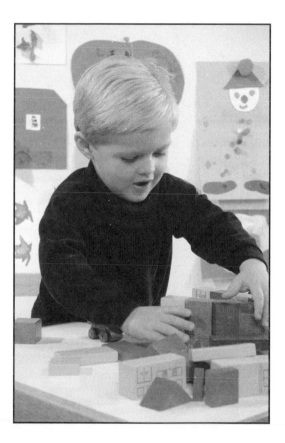

In Sweden preschool children that are allergic to furred pets, as well as other allergens, are placed in special "allergen-avoidance" day-care centers. In these centers, neither children nor staff members are allowed to have furred pets in their homes.

Solving the Pet-Allergy Conundrum

As with other disease-causing allergens, the best advice I can give you is to remove the offender from your home and avoid further exposure at any cost. But I am a realist, and I know that for many of you, getting rid of your pet altogether is not even going to be considered as an option. Of course, if the pet is causing severe discomfort or is responsible for recurrent asthma episodes in you or your children, you really have no choice other than to find the pet another loving home. Sometimes difficult choices need to be made to preserve the health of our loved ones, and surely protecting the health of a child will take precedence when determining whether or not to keep an animal in the home.

If the decision is made to keep the pet, then you should try to create a habitat for the pet that does not include your home and living space. Dogs and cats can be provided with adequate, even luxurious, living accommodations outside of your home. There are many high-quality, insulated, and safe pre-fabricated dog and cat shelters that will protect your pet from the elements and provide a comfortable outdoor habitat. If you absolutely *must* keep your pet indoors, then take steps to create "pet-free" zones in the house where the allergy sufferer can remain free of exposure to the pet-producing allergens. It is particularly beneficial to ensure that bedrooms remain pet free. A high efficiency, high filtration air cleaner should be used in the bedroom, as well as in other areas of the house where pet allergens might affect a sufferer's well-being.

Bathe your pet and wash his or her bedding and toys on a regular basis. Studies show that weekly bathing can reduce the level of allergens produced by pets by as much as 85 percent. Also, take extra steps in your housecleaning. Air-out rooms regularly, vacuum and mop floors, and wipe down your walls to reduce the levels of pet allergen. Change air-conditioner and furnace filters often. You may even want to place a layer of cheesecloth or vent filter over room vents to keep pet hair from being blown about your home.

It is also recommended that you create as close to a fur-and-dander-resistant environment as possible by replacing any carpeting with wood, tile, or vinyl flooring and avoiding the use of upholstered furniture.

If you have pet allergies and have chosen to create completely pet-free environments in your home and office, you could still be exposed to the allergens through the contaminated clothing of visitors. It should not be too much to ask your guests to be sensitive to your allergies. They should avoid handling the pet prior to entering your home or workspace and should take care that pet-contaminated clothing is changed before their visit. Also, if your children are particularly sensitive to pet allergens, talk to school and day-care facility officials. You may even want to consider forming an allergy-watch committee with other parents or your coworkers to educate individuals overseeing the safety of our indoor environments about ways to control the spread of unwelcome pet-produced allergens.

Dogs and cats can be provided with adequate, even luxurious, living accommodations outside of your home.

Nine Steps to Protect Your Premises from Pet Allergens

1. Create a welcoming outside habitat for your pet. Look for safe, insulated, pre-fabricated pet houses that will keep your pet warm and happy and his allergens out of your house!
2. If you *must* keep your pet inside, create "pet-free" zones in the house where the pet is not allowed to go. All bedrooms should be designated pet free.
3. Use a high efficiency, high filtration air cleaner throughout the home and particularly in the bedrooms.
4. Bathe your pet and his bedding and toys on a weekly basis.
5. Thoroughly clean and vacuum your home regularly. Wash down all walls and surfaces and keep bedding clean and free of animal dander.
6. Replace carpeting with wood, vinyl, or tile floors. Get rid of upholstered furniture.
7. Change air conditioner and furnace filters on a regular basis. Place cheesecloth or vent filters over room vents.
8. If you want to maintain a pet-allergen-free home, ask all houseguests to avoid contact with animals prior to visiting your home. Request that they wear only clean, fur-free clothing into your home.
9. Form an allergy-watch committee and educate school, day-care, and office management personnel about ways to avoid pet-allergen contamination of the indoor environment.

CHAPTER 7

Environmental Pollution—What You Don't Know Can Kill You

Hidden Dangers in Your Home

What if there were a ghost or goblin lurking in the shadows of your house? What if there were evil spirits lingering inside your walls, beneath your basement floor, or floating about in the air?

"A ghost or a goblin?" you're probably thinking to yourself. "This man must be mad ... or maybe his years as a surgeon cutting into hearts has finally muddled his brain."

No, I'm not mad. Well, maybe I am just a little crazy about maintaining a healthy quality of life, starting with breathing clean air. What I am about to tell you may alarm you. But please don't dismiss it as the ravings of an overzealous health nut. Believe me when I tell you that my zealous nature has no bearing on the information contained in this chapter. If you are going to seriously tackle the problems of indoor air pollution, you need to be armed with the most important weapon of all—scientifically based information! The dangers I am about to alert you to could be contaminating the air in your home, office, or schoolhouse without your knowing it. They act like invisible ghosts and can be just as damaging as a pack of goblins. You're likely going to need the sleuth-like skills of a ghost-buster to identify and rid your environment of these toxic substances. That's because you can't see them or smell them. They don't make any noise—no screeching sirens are going to go off!—and if you don't take affirmative steps to ferret them out and dispose of them, you are probably not even going to become aware of how sick they are making you and your family until the damage has already been done. I am talking about environmental pollutants—lead, radon, asbestos, and carbon monoxide.

Is There Lead Lurking in Your Lair?

Back before we were aware of its harmful effects, lead was a common component of water pipes and was used as an additive in paint and gasoline, as well as in a variety of other products commonly used to build and decorate our homes, schools, and offices. Even though it is now recognized as a serious environmental pollutant, lead is still present in many older buildings. In fact, it is pretty safe to assume that any structure built before 1978 probably contains levels of lead at an unacceptably high level. Lead is considered to be such a health risk that a decade ago, the United States Secretary of Health and Human Services declared it to be the *number one* environmental threat to children in the country!

Lead-based paint is the most prevalent source of lead exposure today. Harmful exposure levels most often occur in older office buildings or homes where the lead-based paint is exposed or removed by dry scraping, sanding, or open-flame burning. Elevated concentrations of lead particles can also enter your indoor environment in the form of lead dust that is carried in contaminated soil from construction sites, radiator repair shops, or areas where batteries are handled. Airborne lead enters the body when you breathe or swallow lead-contaminated dust particles or water. And the effects can be devastating.

Lead is considered to be such a health risk that a decade ago the United States Secretary of Health and Human Services declared it to be the number one environmental threat to children in the country!

The Environmental Protection Agency reports that 900,000 children ages one to five have dangerously high blood-lead levels. Lead poisoning is particularly prevalent in young children. Babies and toddlers often put their hands and other objects in their mouths, and these objects may have lead on them. In addition, children's growing bodies absorb more lead than adults', and their brains and nervous systems are more sensitive to the damaging effects of lead.

High levels of lead in children can result in slowed growth, behavior and learning problems—such as hyperactivity—hearing problems, damage to the brain and nervous system, and headaches. In adults, elevated lead levels can cause difficulties during pregnancy, reproductive problems, high blood pressure, digestive disorders, nerve disorders, memory and concentration problems, and muscle and joint pain.

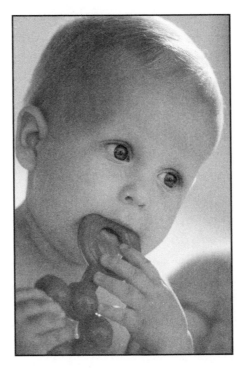

While lead-based paint that is in good condition is not considered a hazard, peeling, chipping, caulking, or cracking lead-based paint can release airborne poisons. If your home has lead-based paint, check the areas that are most likely subject to potential lead-exposing wear and tear: windows and window sills; doors and door frames; stairs, railings, and banisters; and porches and fences. Homes with suspected lead hazards should undergo a risk assessment and paint inspection by qualified experts. Look for specialists that are certified in lead inspection. You might want to start by contacting your state's lead-poisoning prevention program.

If you suspect that your home may have lead paint, then clean up any paint chips immediately. You should also clean floors, windows, and other surfaces weekly. Sponges and mop heads should be thoroughly rinsed after use, and play areas should always be kept clean. The continuous use of a high efficiency, high filtration air cleaner will also assist in the control of airborne lead. If you decide to undergo a lead-removal procedure, it is best to hire a certified lead-abatement contractor to ensure that the job will be done correctly and that all toxic substances are properly removed from the premise.

High levels of lead in children can result in slowed growth, behavior and learning problems, hearing problems, damage to the brain and nervous system, and headaches.

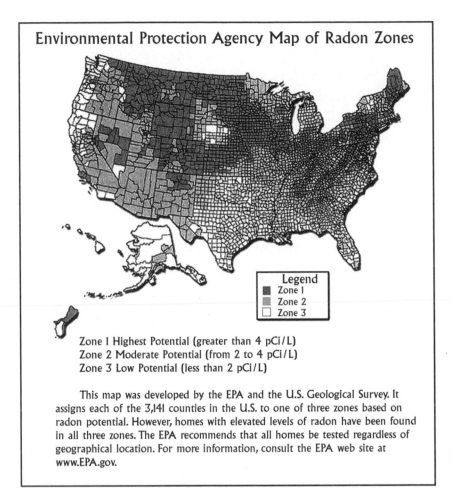

Environmental Protection Agency Map of Radon Zones

Legend
Zone 1
Zone 2
Zone 3

Zone 1 Highest Potential (greater than 4 pCi/L)
Zone 2 Moderate Potential (from 2 to 4 pCi/L)
Zone 3 Low Potential (less than 2 pCi/L)

This map was developed by the EPA and the U.S. Geological Survey. It assigns each of the 3,141 counties in the U.S. to one of three zones based on radon potential. However, homes with elevated levels of radon have been found in all three zones. The EPA recommends that all homes be tested regardless of geographical location. For more information, consult the EPA web site at www.EPA.gov.

The Ravages of Radon

You can't smell radon. You can't see it or taste it either. Its existence does not result from poor habits in hygiene or bad building or decorating decisions. This invisible, odorless, tasteless gas occurs naturally. It comes from the radioactive breakdown of uranium in soil, rock, and water and ends up permeating the air you breathe. It is found all over the United States and can enter a home, school, or office building through cracks in concrete floors and walls, floor drainage, construction joints, and tiny cracks in hollow wall blocks.

Radon is the suspected cause of thousands of deaths each year. The mere act of breathing radon-poisoned air can result in lung cancer. If you combine cigarette smoking with radon inhalation, you are even more likely to develop the deadly disease.

So if the gas is tasteless, odorless, and invisible, how do you know if your home just happens to be built over a radon site? Well, the only way to know for sure is to undergo radon testing. The EPA and the Surgeon General have recommended testing all homes for radon. The EPA has even designated a week in October as National Radon Action Week and has a National Radon Information Line (1-800-767-7236). I cannot emphasize enough the importance of testing. You can call the EPA's national hotline or contact your state's radon center for more information on getting your residence tested. There are even inexpensive self-testing kits that you can purchase at your local home-improvement or hardware store although you are better off using a professional service that has earned accreditation and certification in radon testing. If it turns out that radon is a problem, please seek a qualified expert to mitigate the effects of radon in your indoor environment.

Radon is the suspected cause for thousands of deaths each year. The mere act of breathing radon-poisoned air can result in lung cancer.

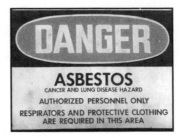

Take Up Arms Against Asbestos

Y ou've probably heard people talk about asbestos. Lawsuits concerning asbestos abound, and people often worry that their office buildings or children's schools contain the substance. But what exactly is asbestos? Do you have it in *your* home, school, and office? And if so, can it really hurt you?

Asbestos is the name given to a group of natural minerals that form masses of fibers that can be separated into threads. These threads have historically been added to products to strengthen them, primarily in building materials because they provide fire resistance and heat insulation. Asbestos has been used since the late nineteenth century and is still in use today. In the late 1970s, the federal government banned the use of asbestos in certain building materials because of the excessive amounts of asbestos fiber that were released into the environment. It was discovered that people who breathe high levels of this particulate matter have a high risk of coming down with life-threatening illnesses. In fact, while studies have concluded that high levels of asbestos exposure are hazardous, the EPA has concluded that there is, in fact, no safe level of exposure to asbestos fibers. Asbestos is still being used in construction materials, for shipbuilding, and by the automotive industry, but its use has been steadily declining over the past thirty years.

Asbestos is only dangerous if it becomes airborne. Most of the time, if a building contains asbestos, it will not cause a problem unless there is crumbling or flaking of the material. It is usually safer to leave asbestos in place than to have it removed by someone who is not specially trained in handling the product.

People breathing high levels of asbestos are at great risk of developing mesthelioma, a malignancy of the lining of the chest and peritoneal cavities, and asbestosis, an intense scarring of the lungs. Lung cancer can also result from exposure to asbestos, particularly when the individual has also been a cigarette smoker.

So, back to our initial questions. Do the buildings you work in and live in contain asbestos? Probably. Do you have cause for concern? It depends. If there is *any* damage or deterioration in asbestos-containing materials, you could indeed be in danger. It is best to contact a trained asbestos specialist to inspect any suspected exposed asbestos, and if a problem is encountered, only a skilled professional should remove the offending material. If you think you have been exposed to asbestos, you should consult a health professional immediately, especially if you are experiencing respiratory symptoms.

While studies have concluded that high levels of asbestos exposure are hazardous, the EPA has concluded that there is, in fact, no safe level of exposure for asbestos fibers.

Is Your Home Leaking Lethal Gas?

It can enter your home at any time, and you won't even know that it is there. You may become confused, nauseous, dizzy, and short of breath. You may feel a headache coming on or start feeling faint. Maybe you decide to lie down for a while, thinking that you are coming down with the flu or are experiencing a mild bout of food poisoning. If you are not well versed in the signs of carbon monoxide poisoning and do not immediately get outside to fresh air, you could even die.

Carbon monoxide is odorless. It is colorless. And it is deadly. A gas that is produced by the incomplete combustion

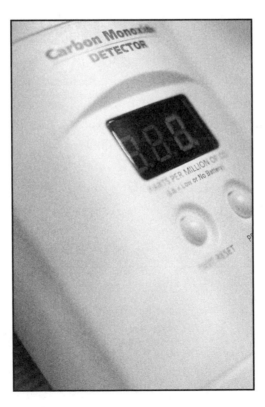

of carbon-containing products and fuels such as wood, natural gas, gasoline, and other petroleum products, carbon monoxide brings on a silent death. By inhaling carbon monoxide, you deprive your body and your brain of oxygen. And so you suffocate, often in your sleep.

Because carbon monoxide is almost impossible to detect, and because the symptoms mimic other illnesses, prevention is the key to avoiding carbon monoxide poisoning. All furnaces and combustible heaters should be checked each year *before* firing them up for the winter season. A malfunctioning heating unit can cause the production of toxic levels of carbon monoxide.

Whenever possible, you should purchase appliances that vent fumes to the outside. Have them professionally installed and make sure they are properly maintained according to the manufacturer's instructions. *Never* idle a car in a garage— even if the garage door is open. A high concentration of fumes can build up in a short amount of time. The fumes can even make their way into your home. *Never* use a gas oven to heat your home or use a charcoal grill indoors. And *don't ignore* symptoms of carbon monoxide poisoning! The minute you feel short of breath, nauseous, headaches, mental confusion, dizzy, or faint, go outside for fresh air! If the symptoms persist, then go to the hospital and tell the health-care professionals that you suspect carbon monoxide poisoning.

It is a good idea to install a carbon monoxide detector— a device much like a smoke detector—in your home. However, carbon monoxide detectors should never be your sole defense against carbon monoxide poisoning. While they can serve as a good backup, these detectors are not always reliable. As previously stated, prevention through proper maintenance of potentially hazardous appliances and furnaces is your best defense against carbon monoxide poisoning.

A gas that is produced by the incomplete combustion of carbon-containing products and fuels such as wood, natural gas, gasoline, and other petroleum products, carbon monoxide brings on a silent death. By inhaling carbon monoxide, you deprive your body and your brain of oxygen. And so you suffocate, often in your sleep.

Twelve Steps to Fighting Environmental Pollution

1. Check your home for the existence of lead paint. Inspect for any chipping paint around doors, windows, stairs, railings, porches, and banisters.
2. If you suspect that you have lead paint, clean up paint chips and thoroughly clean floors, windows, and other surfaces and have your home inspected by a qualified lead specialist.
3. Hire a qualified lead-abatement contractor to remove dangerous lead from your home.
4. Have your home tested for radon, preferably by a qualified expert.
5. Inspect your home for deterioration in or damage to asbestos-containing materials.
6. Never expose or remove asbestos-laden materials on your own. Use the services of a qualified asbestos expert.
7. Consult a health professional if you think you may have been exposed to airborne asbestos.
8. Inspect all furnaces and combustible heaters each year to ensure that they are functioning properly and not emitting carbon monoxide.
9. Purchase and install appliances that vent fumes to the outside.
10. Never idle a car in your garage—even if the door is kept open.
11. If you feel *any* symptoms of carbon monoxide poisoning, immediately get to fresh air and consult a health-care professional.
12. Install a carbon monoxide detector in your home.

SOME RECOMMENDATIONS TO HELP YOU CLEAR THE AIR AND BREATHE EASIER

Throughout this book, I've attempted to offer concrete suggestions for improving your indoor environment so that you and your family can clear the air and enjoy a better quality of life....with every breath you take. The following is a list of products that I have found particularly useful in creating a safer and allergy-free (or at least allergy-reduced) indoor environment. Additional products can be found by contacting Health-Mor At Home: 1-800-662-2471 or by accessing their web page: www.filterqueen.com.

Dust mask: When working outdoors or cleaning inside, using quality dust masks can help protect you from dust, pollen and other allergens. High efficiency masks (such as the 3M® 8210 or 8233 Particulate Respirator) have proven particularly effective in protecting against unwanted microscopic allergens.

Allergy-free bed pillows and bedding: By replacing conventional pillows with allergy-resistant fiber-laden bed pillows, you can greatly reduce your bedtime exposure to allergens. I recommend the Allersoft™ pillows. These state-of-the art pillows utilize advance weaving technology to produce a tightly woven material that is air breathable and water vapor transmittive. Wash the pillows regularly in hot water and vacuum them with the Filter Queen® home cleaning system (see below). I also recommend Health-Mor at Home Encasings for your pillows, mattresses, and box springs.

Air cleaners: I have found the Filter Queen® Medical Recirculating Air Cleaner and the Acclero™ brand air cleaner to be particularly effective in keeping indoor air clean and healthy. These systems boast filtration levels of 99.98% at 0.1 micron, which is better than ordinary HEPA filtration systems, and are proven to clear your air of even the smallest air polluting particles of dust, pollen, smoke, animal dander, mold spores, harmful fibers, and other air polluting substances. Also, the exhausts are on the top so the systems don't blow floor and carpeting dust around your indoor environment the way conventional air filtration systems do. Another distinguishing characteristic is the mechanical air filters used in these products do not produce ozone, a respiratory irritant.

Humidity control: Because humidity plays such an integral part in the proliferation of mold and other allergy-producing organisms, gauging the level of humidity in your home is crucial in the fight against mold. The Honeywell® Humidity Gauge displays the humidity level and room temperature so that you can be sure that your home is not a welcoming environment for humidity-hungry pollutants.

Home cleaning system: Because standard vacuum cleaners can actually exacerbate the spread of allergens, I highly recommend replacing conventional home cleaning systems with the Filter Queen® home care surface cleaner system. By incorporating a five-stage filtration system, dirt, dust mites, allergens, germs, gases, and odors are actually captured and removed from the environment. The Filter Queen® system has a 99.98% filter efficiency at 0.1 micron, which exceeds standards set for HEPA filtration and maintains air flow during its use.

Carbon monoxide detectors: Because carbon monoxide is an odorless invisible and deadly gas, every home should have a carbon monoxide detector. First Alert® makes a variety of detectors – battery powered, combination carbon monoxide/smoke detector – for the home.

Vent filters: Vent filters help stop dust and other allergens from entering your home. Look for vent filters that are made of highly efficient fibers that collect airborne particles.

Definitions

Airway Hyper Responsiveness (AHR) — A constrictive condition that occurs in the airways of the lungs during an asthma attack.

Allergen — An antigenic substance capable of producing immediate-type hypersensitivity reaction by the immune system.

Allergic Reaction — Inappropriate or exaggerated reaction of the immune system to certain substances.

Allergy Immunotherapy ("allergy shots") — This involves giving incremental increasing doses of the substance to which a person is allergic.

Animal Dander — The skin particles that flake off from an animal's skin.

Antigen — Any substance that is capable of inducing specific immune response.

Asthma — A respiratory condition marked by recurrent attacks of paroxysmal dyspnea and associated wheezing.

Atopy — A genetic predisposition toward the development of environmental antigens.

Autoimmune Disease — A disturbance of the immune system whereby an individual develops an allergy to a specific organ or product of that organ.

Biological Pollutants — Living organisms that are harmful as allergens or invaders of the human body.

Building-Related Illness — Specific illnesses that occur directly as exposure to certain building products.

Carbon Monoxide — Dangerous gas that results from incomplete combustion of fossil fuels.

Dust Mite (ACARID) — Microscopic arthropod that is highly allergenic and lives in mattresses, pillows, carpets, and upholstered furniture and feeds off human/animal dander.

Fungi — A major group of saprophytic and parasitic asexual lower plants that lack chlorophyll and include molds, yeasts, rusts, mildews, and mushrooms.

Glucans — Substances that are part of the cell walls of molds. They activate the human immune system, and many people believe that **glucans** are the cause of non-specific health complaints of **sick-building syndrome**.

HEPA — Technology developed by U.S. Atomic Energy Commission to remove airborne/radioactive particles. A true HEPA filter must be capable of removing 99.97 percent of particles as small as 0.3 microns.

Humidifier Fever — A respiratory infection that occurs from breathing mist from a humidifier that is contaminated with microbiological contamination.

Immunoglobulin E — An antibody that is formed in response to an allergic challenge to the immune system.

Inhalant — A substance taken into the body by way of the nose, trachea, or other parts of the respiratory system.

Mold Spores — Reproductive portion of mold.

Sick-Building Syndrome — Occurs when a substantial group of individuals in a building or location in a building complains of a diffuse but common set of complaints relating to illness.

T-Cell Immunodysfunction — Impairment of the immune system when the T-cell portion is unable to respond properly.

Volatile Organic Compounds (VOC) — These are organic compounds with melting points below room temperature. Gasoline, certain home furnishings, and products used for cleaning that emit volatile organic compounds into the air.

References

Abbott J, Cameron J, Taylor B. House dust mite counts in different types of mattresses, sheepskins and carpets, and a comparison of brushing and vacuuming methods. *Clin Allergy* 1981; 11:589–95.

Allergy and Asthma Network.

American Academy of Allergy & Immunology.

American Academy of Allergy, Asthma and Immunology.

American College of Allergy & Immunology.

American Conference of Governmental Industrial Hygienists (ACGIH) (1998). Threshold Limit Values for Chemical Substances and Physical Agents and Biological Exposure Indices 1998, Cincinnati, OH.

American Lung Association, Air Quality, State of the Air: 2000.

American Lung Association of D.C.: 202/682-5864; web site www.aladc.org/.

American Lung Association of Minnesota. Health House http://www.healthhouse.org.

American Lung Association, et al. Indoor air pollution: an introduction for health professionals. U.S EPA Internet site at http://www.epa.gov/iedweb00/pubs/ hpguide.html accessed on 22 January 1998.

American Lung Association. When you can't breathe, nothing else matters: the truth about indoor air. American Lung Association Internet site at http://www.lungusa.org/noframes/global/news/association/asnthetruth.html accessed on 14 April 1998.

Andriessen JW, Brunekreef B, Roemer W. Home dampness and respiratory health status in European children. *Clin Exp Allergy* 1998;28:1191–200.

Anonymous. Position statement. Environmental allergen avoidance in allergic asthma. Ad Hoc Working Group on Environmental Allergens and Asthma. [Review] [45 refs] *Journal of Allergy & Clinical Immunology* 103(2 Pt 1):203–5, 1999 Feb.

Arlian LG. Biology and ecology of house dust mites, Dermatophagoides spp. And Euroglyphus spp. *Immunol Allergy Clin North Am* 1989; 9 (2):339–56.

Arlian LG, Bernstein D, Bernstein IL, et al. Prevalence of dust mites in the homes of people with asthma living in eight different geographic areas of the U.S. *J Allergy Clin Immunol* 1992;90:292–300.

Arruda LK, Vailes LD, Mann BJ, Shannon J, Fox JW, Vedvick TS, et al. Molecular cloning of a major cockroach (Blattella germanica) allergen, Bla g 2: sequence homology to the aspartic proteases. *J Biol Chem* 1995; 270:19563–8.

Asthma & Allergy Foundation of America.

Bergmann R, Woodcock A. Whole population or high risk group? Childhood asthma. *Eur Respir J* 1998:27(Suppl):9–12s.

Berry RW, Brown VM, Coward SKD, Crump DR, Gavin M, Grimes CP, et al. Indoor air quality in homes. The Building Research Establishment Indoor Environment Study. BRE Report 1996. London: Construction Research Communications; 1996.

Bierbaun P, Gorman R, Wallingford K. The NIOSH Approach to Conducting Indoor Air Quality Investigations in Office Buildings. Energy Tech no. 16 (9):347–61 (1989).

Bjorksten B, Holt BJ, Baron-Hay MJ, Munir AK, Holt PG. Low-level exposure to house dust mites stimulates T-cell responses during early childhood independent of atopy. *Clin Exp Allergy* 1996;26:775–9.

Bollinger ME, Eggleston PA, Flanagan E, Wood RA. Cat antigen in homes with and without cats may induce allergic symptoms. *J Allergy Clin Immunol* 1996; 97:907–14.

Boulet LP, Cartier A, Thompson NC, et al. Asthma and increases in non allergic bronchial responsiveness from seasonal pollen exposure. *J Allergy Clin Immunol* 1983;71:399–406.

Burge H, Hoyer M. Indoor Air Quality. *Appl Occup Environ Hyg* 5(2):84–93(1990).

Burr ML, Butland BK, King S, et al. Changes in asthma prevalence: two surveys 15 years apart. *Arch Dis Child* 1988;64:1452–8.

Call RS, Smith TF, Morris E, Chapman M, Platts-Mills TAE. Risk factors for asthma in inner city children. *J Pediatr* 1992;121:862–6.

Chan-Yeung M, Becker A, Lam J, Dimich-Ward H, Ferguson A, Warren P, et al. House dust mite allergen levels in two cities in Canada: effects of season, humidity, city and home characteristics. *Clin Exp Allergy* 1995;25:240–6.

Chapman MD. Cockroach allergens: a common cause of asthma in North American cities. *Insights Allergy* 1993;8:1–8.

Charpin D, Birnbaum J, Haddi E, et al. Altitude and allergy to house dust mites: a paradigm of the influence of environmental exposure on allergic sensitization. *Am Rev Respir Dis* 1991;143:983–6.

Colloff MD. Mites from house dust in Glasgow. *Med Vet Entomol* 1987;1:163–8.

Croner S, Kjellman NI. Natural history of bronchial asthma in childhood: a prospective study from birth up to 12–14 years of age. *Allergy* 1992;47(Suppl):150–7.

Custovic A, Green R, Fletcher A, Smith A, Pickering CAC, Chapman MD, Woodcock A. Aerodynamic properties of the major dog allergen, Can f 1:distribution in homes, concentration and particle size of allergen in the air. *Am J Crit Care Med* 1996. In press.

Custovic A, Taggart SCO, Francis HC, et al. Exposure to house dust mite allergens and the clinical activity of asthma. *J Allergy Clin Immunol* 1996; 98:64–72.

Custovic A, Taggart SCO, Kennaugh JH, Woodcock AA. Portable dehumidifiers in the control of house dust mites and mite allergens. *Clin Exp Allergy* 1995;25:312–6.

Custovic A, Woodcock A. Indoor environmental factors and respiratory illness (editorial; comment). *Clinical & Experimental Allergy.* 28(10):1178–81, 1998 Oct.

Cybendal T, Vik H, Elsayed S. Dust from carpeted and smooth floors. *Allergy* 1989;44:401–11.

D.C. Environmental Health Administration Division of Air Quality:202/535–2.

D.C. Office of Occupational Health and Safety:202/787-4160.

De Blay F, Chapman MD, Platts-Mills, TAE. Airborne cat allergen (Fel d 1): environmental control with the cat in situ. *Am Rev Respir Dis* 1991;143:1334–9.

De Blay F, Sanchez J, Hedelin G, Perez-Infante A, Verot A, Chapman M, Pauli G. Dust and airborne exposure to allergens derived from cockroach (Blatella germanica) in low-cost public housing in Strasbourg (France). *Journal of Allergy & Clinical Immunology.* 99(1 Pt 1):107–12, 1997 Jan.

De Boer R. The control of house dust mite allergens in rugs. *J Allergy Clin Immunol* 1990;86:808–14.

———. Movements of house dust mites in response to changing physical circumstances. *Proc Exp Appl Entomol* NEV Amsterdam 1996;7:247–8.

———. Reflections on the control of mites and mite allergens. *Allergy* 1998; 53.

De Boer R, Kuller K. Mattresses as a winter refuge for house dust mites. *Allergy* 1997;52:299–305.

Dingle, Peter, Murdock University WA Research Findings.

Dotterud LK, Van TD, Kvammen B, et al. Alleren content in dust from homes and schools in northern Norway in relation to sensitization and allergy symptoms in schoolchildren. *Clin Exp Allergy* 1997; 27:252–61.

Eggleston PA, Wood RA, Rand C, Nixon W, Chen P, Lukk P. Removal of cockroach allergen from inner-city homes. *Journal of Allergy & Clinical Immunology* 104(4 Pt 1):842–6, 1999 Oct.

Ehnert B, Lau-Schadendorf S, Weber A, Buettner P, Schou C, Wahn U. Reducing domestic exposure to dust mite allergen reduces bronchial hyperreactivity in sensitive children with asthma. *J Allergy Clin Immunol* 1992;90:135–8.

Einarsson R, Munir AKM, Dreborg SKG. Allergens in school dust. II. Major mite (Der p I, Der f I) allergens in dust from Swedish schools. *J Allergy Clin Immunol* 1995;95:1049–53.

Ellul-Micallef Al-Ali S. The spectrum of bronchial asthma in Kuwait. *Clin Allergy* 1994; 14:509–17.

Enberg RN, Shamie SM, McCullough J, Ownby DR. Ubiquitous presence of cat allergen in cat-free buildings:probable dispersal from human clothing. *Ann Allergy* 1993;70:471–4.

Environmental Protection Agency. Building air quality: A guide for building owners and facility managers.

————. Indoor air facts no. 4: Sick building syndrome. April 1991.

Epton MJ, Martin IR, Graham P, Healy PE, Smith H, Balasubramaniam R, Harvey IC, Fountain DW, Hedley J, Town GI. Climate and aeroallergen levels in asthma: a 12 month prospective study. *Thorax.* 52(6):528–34, 1997 Jun.

Finn P MD, Boudreau J, He H MD, Wang Y MD, Chapman M MD, Vincent C PhD, Burge H PhD, Weiss S MD, Perkins D MD, Gold D MD. Children at risk for asthma: Home allergen levels, lymphocyte proliferation, and wheeze. *J Allergy Clin Immunol* Vol 105:5.

Flannery EM, Herbison GP, Hewitt CJ, Holdaway MD, Jones DT, Sears MR. Sheepskins and bedding in childhood, and the risk of development of bronchial asthma. *Aust NZ J Med* 1994;24:687–92.

Fletcher AM, Pickering CAC, Custovic A, Simpson J, Kennaugh J, Woodcock A. Reduction in humidity as a method of controlling mites and mite allergens: the use of mechanical ventilation in British domestic dwellings. *Clin Exp Allergy* 1996;26:1051–6.

Garrett MH, Rayment PR, Hooper MA, et al. Indoor airborne fungal spores, house dampness and associations with environmental factors and respiratory health in children. *Clin Exp Allergy* 1998; 28:459–67.

Gelber LE, Seltzer LH, Bouzoukis JK, Pollart SM, Chapman D, Platts-Mills TAE. Sensitization and exposure to indoor allergens as risk factors for asthma among patients presenting to hospital. *Am Rev Respir Dis* 1993;147:573–8.

Gergen PJ, Mortimer KM, Eggleston P, Rosenstreich D, Mitchell H, Ownby D, Kattan M, Baker D, Wright EC, Slavin R, Malveaux F. Results of the National Cooperative Inner-City Asthma Study (NCICAS) environmental intervention to reduce cockroach allergen exposure in inner-city homes. *Journal of Allergy & Clinical Immunology,* 103(3 Pt 1):501–6, 1999 Mar.

Halonen M, Stern DA, Wright AL, et al. Alternaria as the major allergen for asthma in children raised in a desert environment. *Am J Respir Crit Care Med* 1997; 155:1356–61.

Hart BJ, Whitehead L. Ecology of house dust mites in Oxfordshire. *Clin Exp Allergy* 1990;20:203–9.

Hasnain SM, Wilson JD, Newhook FJ. Fungi and disease. Fungal allergy and respiratory disease. *NZ Med J* 1985;98:342–6.

Hayden ML, Rose G, Diduch KB, et al. Benzyl benzoate moist powder: investigation of acaricidal activity in cultures and reduction of dust mite allergens in carpets. *J Allergy Clin Immunol* 1992;89:536–45.

Hegarty JM, Rouhbakhsh S, Warner JA, Warner JO. A comparison of the effect of conventional and filter vacuum cleaners on airborne house dust mite allergen. *Respir Med* 1995;89:279–84.

Hiipakka DW, Buffington JR. Resolution of sick building syndrome in a high security facility. *Appl Occup Environ Hyg* 2000 Aug;15(8):635–43

Hill DJ, Thompson PJ, Stewart GA, et al. The Melbourne house dust mite study: eliminating house dust mites in the domestic environment. *J Allergy Clin Immunol* 1997;99:323–9.

Holgate ST. Asthma: a dynamic disease of inflammation and repair. *Ciba Found Symp* 1997;206:5–34, 106–10.

Ichikawa K, Iwasaki E, Baba M, Chapman MD. High prevalence of sensitization to cat allergen among Japanese children with asthma, living without cats. *Clin Exp Allergy* 1999;29:754–61.

Kalra Owen SJ, Hepworth J, Woodcock A. Airborne house dust mite antigen after vacuum cleaning. *Lancet* 1990;336:449.

Kalra S, Crank P, Hepworth J, Pickering CAC, Woodcock A. Absence of seasonal variation in concentrations of the house dust mite allergen Der p 1 in South Manchester homes. *Thorax* 1992; 47:928–31.

Kang B. Study on cockroach antigen as a probable causative agent in bronchial asthma. *J Allergy Clin Immunol* 1976;58:357–65.

Kang B, Wu CW, Johnson J. Characteristics and diagnoses of cockroach sensitive bronchial asthma. *Ann Allergy* 1992;68:237–44.

Korsgaard J. House dust mites and absolute indoor humidity. *Allergy* 1983;38:85–92.

———. Mechanical ventilation and house dust mites: a controlled investigation. In: Van Moerbeke D, editor. *Dust Mite Allergens and Asthma*. Brussles:UCB Institute of Allergy; 1991.p87–9.

———. Mite asthma and residency: a case-control study on the impact of exposure to house-dust mites in dwellings. *Am Rev Respir Dis* 1983;128:231–5.

———. Preventive measures in mite asthma. A controlled trial. *Allergy* 1983;38:93–102.

Li CY, Hsu LY. Home dampness and childhood respiratory symptoms in subtropical climate. *Arch Environ Health* 1996; 51:42–6.

Lin RY, LaFrance J, Sauter D. Hypersensitivity to common indoor aeroallergens in asthmatic patients. *Ann Allergy* 1993;71:33–9.

Luczynska CM, Li Y, Chapman MD, Platts-Mills, TAE. Airborne concentrations and particle size distribution of allergen derived from domestic cats (Felis domesticus). *Am Rev Respir Dis* 1990;141:361–7.

Marbury MC, Woods JE. Building-related illnesses. In Samet J., Spengler J, eds. *Indoor Air Pollution: A Health Perspective*. Baltimore: Johns Hopkins Univ. Press, 1991, pp. 319–20.

Marks GB, Tovey ER, Green W, et al. The effect of changes in house dust mite allergen exposure on the severity of asthma. *Clin Exp Allergy* 1995; 25:114–8.

Martin IR, Henwood JL, Wilson F, Koning MM, Pike AJ, Smith S, Town GI. House dust mite and cat allergen levels in domestic dwellings in Christchurch. *New Zealand Medical Journal.* 110(1046):229–31, 1997 Jun 27.

Martinez FD, Wright AL, Taussig LM, Holberg CJ, Halonen M, Morgan Medical Associates. *N Engl J Med* 1995; 332:133–8.

Maryland Department of Labor, Licensing & Regulation. Indoor Air Quality.

Meijer GG, Postma DS, Von der Heide S, et al. Exogenous stimuli and circadian peak expiratory flow variation in allergic asthmatic children. *Am J Respir Crit Care Med* 1996; 153:237–42.

Merrett TG, Pantin CFA, Dimand AH, Merrett J. Screening for IgE mediated allergy. *Allergy* 1980;35:491–501

Mitchell EA. Increasing prevalence of asthma in children. *NZ Med J* 1983; 96:463–4.

Mitchell EB, Wilkins SR, McCallum Deighton J, Platts-Mills, TAE. Reduction of house dust mite allergen levels in the home: use of the acaricide, pirimiphos methyl. *Clin Allergy* 1985;15:235–40.

Miyazawa H, Sakaguchi M, Inouye S, Ikeda K, Honbo Y, Yasueda H, et al. Seasonal changes in mite allergen (Der I and Der II) concentrations in Japanese homes. *Ann Allergy Asthma Immunol* 1996; 76:170–4.

Morrow-Brown H, Merrett TG. Effectiveness of an acaricide in management of house dust mite allergy. *Ann Allergy* 1991;67:25–31.

Mosbech H, Jensen A, Heinig JH, Schou C. House dust mite allergens on different types of mattresses. *Clin Exp Allergy* 1991; 21:351–5.

Moyes CD, Waldon J, Ramada D, Crane J, Pearce N. Respiratory symptoms and environmental factors in schoolchildren in the Bay of Plenty. *NZ Med J* 1995; 108: 358–61.

Munir AKM, Bjorksten B, Einarsson R, et al. Mite allergens in relation to home conditions and sensitization of asthmatic children from three climatic regions. *Allergy* 1995;50:55–64.

Munir AKM, Einarsson R, Dreborg SKG. Vacuum cleaning decreased the levels of mite allergens in house dust. *Pediatr Allergy Immunol* 1993;4:136–43.

Munir AKM, Kjellman NIM, Bjorksten B. Exposure to indoor allergens in early infancy and sensitization. *J Allergy Clin Immunol* 1997;100:177–81.

Murray AB, Zuk P. The seasonal variation in a population of house dust mites in a North American city. *J Allergy Clin Immunol* 1979; 64:266–9.

National Asthma Education Program. Guidelines for the diagnosis and management of asthma. National Institutes of Health; July 1997; DHHS NIH Pub no. 97-4051.

National Institute of Environmental Health Sciences. Headline Watch: Bedding and asthma, allergies.

National Lead Information Center.

National Radon Hotline.

Niven R, Fletcher AM, Pickering AC, Custovic A, Sivour JB, Preece AR, Oldham L, Francis HC. Attempting to control mite allergens with mechanical ventilation and dehumidification in British houses. *Journal of Allergy & Clinical Immunology* 103(5 Pt 1):756–62, 1999 May.

Norback D, Michael I, Widstrom J. Indoor air quality and personnel factors related to the sick building syndrome. Seand. *J. Work Environ Health* 16(2):121–28 (1990).

O'Hallaren MT, Yunginger JW, Offord KP, et al. Exposure to an aeroallergen as a possible precipitating factor in respiratory arrest in young patients with asthma. *N Engl J Med* 1991;324:359–63.

Oner AL, Bodini A, Piacentini GL. Environmental allergens and childhood asthma. [Review] [67 refs] *Clinical & Experimental Allergy* 28 Suppl 5:76–81, 1998 Nov.

Parrott K.Virginia Polytechnic Institute and State University indoor air quality: Reducing health risks and improving the air you breathe.

Parvaneh S, Kronqvist M, Johansson E, van Hage-Hamsten M. Exposure to an abundance of cat (Fel d 1) and dog (Can f 1) allergens in Swedish farming households. *Allergy* 1999;54:229–34.

Patchett KL, Lewis S, Wickens K, Crane J, Fitzharris P. Fel d I levels in Wellington primary schools and on children's clothing. *J Allergy Clin Immunol* 1996;97:A957.

Peat JK, Salome CM, Woolcock AJ. Longitudinal changes in atopy during a 4 year period: relation to bronchial hyperresponsiveness and respiratory symptoms in a population sample of Australian schoolchildren. *J Allergy Clin Immunol* 1990; 85:65–74.

Peat JK, Tovey E, Toelle BG, Haby MM, Gray EJ, Mahmic A, et al. Asthma severity and morbidity in a population sample of Sydney schoolchildren: Part II. Importance of house dust mite allergens. *Aust NZ J Med* 1994; 24:370–76.

———. House dust mite allergens: a major risk factor for childhood asthma in Australia.*Am J Respir Crit Care Med* 1996;153:141–6.

Peroni D, Piacentini GL, Boner AL. The effects of antigen avoidance at high altitude in allergic asthmatic children. *Aci Int* 1996; 8:151–4.

Platts-Mills, TA, Chapman MD. Dust mites:immunology, allergic disease, and environmental control. *J Allergy Clin Immunol* 1987;80:755–75.

Platts-Mills, TA, deWeck AL. Dust mite allergens and asthma-a world wide problem. *J Allergy Clin Immunol* 1989;83:416–27.

Platts-Mills, TA, Hayden M, Chapman MD, Wilkins SR. Seasonal variation in dust mite and grass-pollen allergens in dust from the houses of patients with asthma. *J Allergy Clin Immunol* 1987; 79:781–91.

Platts-Mills TA, Sporik RB, Chapman MD, Heymann PW. The role of domestic allergens. *Ciba Found Symp* 1997;206:173–89.

Platts-Mills, TAE. How environment affects patients with allergic disease: Indoor allergens and asthma. *Ann allergy* 1994;72:381–4.

Platts-Mills, TAE, Tovey ER, Mitchell EB, et al. Reduction of bronchial hyperreactivity following prolonged allergen avoidance. *Lancet* 1982, ii:675–8.

Platts-Mills, TAE, Vervolet D, Thomas WR, Aalberse RC, Chapman MD. Dust mite allergens and asthma: report of the Third International Workshop. *J Allergy Clin Immunol* 1997;100:S1–S24.

Platts-Mill TAE, Vervloet D, Wayne RT, et al. Indoor allergens and asthma. Report of the Third International Workshop. *J Allergy Clin Immunol* 1997; 100:S1–S24.

Pollart SM, Smith TF, Morris EC, Gelber LE, Platts-Mills, TA, Chapman MD. Environmental exposure to cockroach allergens: analysis with monoclonal antibody based enzyme immunoassays. *J Allergy Clin Immunol* 1991;87:505–10.

Prescott SL, Macaubas C, Smallacombe T, Holt BJ, Sly PD, Holt PG. Development of allergen-specific T-cell memory in atopic and normal children. *Lancet* 1999;353:196–200.

Rak S. Effects of immunotherapy on the inflammation in pollen asthma. *Allergy* 1993; 48:125–8.

Raunio P, Pasanen AL, Reiman M, Virtanen T. Cat, dog, and house dust mite allergen levels of house dust in Finnish apartments. *Allergy* 1998:53:195–99. Munksgaard 1998.

Reid BL, Bennett GW. Apartments: field trials of abamectin bait formulations. *Insecticide Acaracide Tests* 1989;17:4.

Rosenstreich DL, Eggleston P, Kattan M, Baker D, Slavin RG, Gergen P, et al. The role of cockroach allergy and exposure to cockroach allergen in causing morbidity among inner-city children with asthma. *N Engl J Med* 1997;336:1356–63.

Rostron J, Introduction. In Rostron, J, editor. *Sick Building Syndrome: Concepts, Issues and Practice.* London: E & FN Spon, 1997, p.1.

Rowntree S, Cogswell JJ, Platts-Mills, TAE, et al. Development of IgE and IgG antibodies to food and inhalant allergens in children at risk of atopic disease. *Arch Dis Child* 1985;60:727–35.

Sakaguchi M, Inouye S, Irie T, Miyazawa H, Watanabe M, Yasueada H, et al. Airborne cat (Fel d 1), dog (Can f 1), and mite (Der 1 and Der 2) allergen levels in the homes of Japan. *J Allergy Clin Immunol* 1993;92:797–802.

Sarpong SB, Hamilton RG, Eggleston PA, Adkinson NF Jr. Socio-economic status and race as risk factors for cockroach allergen exposure and sensitization in children with asthma. *J Allergy Clin Immunol* 1996;97:1393–401.

Sarpong SB, Karrison T. Season of birth and cockroach allergen sensitization in children with asthma. [published erratum appears in *J Allergy Clin Immunol* 1998 Sep;102(3):448]. *Journal of Allergy & Clinical Immunology* 101(4 Pt 1):566–8, 1998 Apr.

Sarpong SB, Wood RA, Eggleston PA. Short term effects of extermination and cleaning on cockroach allergen Bla g 2 in settled dust. *Ann Allergy Asthma Immunol* 1996;76:257–60.

Sawyer G, Tohill S, Shaw R, et al. Investigation of house dust mite load in sheepskins used in infant bedding. (Abstr) *Aust NZ J Med* 1997:27:233.

Shaw R, Crane J, O'Donnell TV, Porteous LE, Coleman ED. Increasing asthma prevalence in a rural New Zealand adolescent population: 1975-89. *Arch Dis Child* 1990; 65:1319–23.

Sheffer AL (chairman) for the International Asthma management Project. International consensus report on diagnosis and treatment of asthma. *Eur Respir J* 1992;5:601–41.

Smedje G, Norback D, Edling C. Asthma among secondary schoolchildren in relation to the school environment. *Clin Exp Allergy* 1997;27:1270–8.

Solomon WR, Platts-Mills, TAE. Aerobiology of inhalant allergens. In: Middleton E Jr, Reed CE, Ellis EF, Adkinson NF Jr, Yunginger JW, Busse WW, editors. *Allergy: Principles and Practice.* 4th ed St. Louis: Mosby; 1993. p.469–528.

Sporik R, Holgate S, Platts-Mills TAE, Cogswell J. Exposure to house dust mite allergen (der p 1) and the development of asthma in childhood. *N Eng J Med* 1990;323:502–7.

Sporik R, Ingram JM, Price W, Sussman JH, Honsinger RW, Platts-Mills, TA. Association of asthma with serum IgE and skin test reactivity to allergens among children living at high altitude: tickling the dragon's breath. *Am J Respir Crit Care Med* 1995;151:1388–92.

Sporik R, Platts-Mills, TAE, Cogswell JJ. Exposure to house dust mite allergen of children admitted to hospital with asthma. *Clin Exp Allergy* 1993;23:740–6.

Stephen FR, McIntyre DA, Lane A, Raw GJ, Wiech CR, Frederick JM. Ventilation and house air tightness:effect on indoor temperature and humidity in Southampton, UK. *Building Serv Eng Res Technol* 1997;18:141–7.

Stewart GA. The molecular biology of allergens. In Busse WW, Holgate ST, editors. *Asthma and Rhinitis.* Boston: Blackwell; 1995. p. 898–932.

Strachan DP. Is allergic disease programmed in early life? *Clin Exp Allergy* 1994;24:603–5.

Targonski PV, Persky VW, Ramekrishnan V. Effect of environmental molds on risk of death from asthma during the pollen season. *J Allergy Clin Immunol* 1995;95:955–61.

Task Group on Lung Dynamics. Deposition and retention models for internal dosimetry of the human respiration tract. *Health Physics* 1966;12:173–207.

Tovey ER, Chapman MD, Wells CW, Platts-Mills TAE. The distribution of dust mite allergen in houses of patients with asthma. *Am Rev Respir Dis* 1981;124:630–5.

United States Consumer Product Safety Commission, Washington, D.D. 20207, for copies of Humidifier Safety Alert.

United States Department of Housing and Urban Development's Healthy Home Program.

United States Department of Labor, Occupational Safety and Health Administration, OSHA: Proposed standard for indoor air quality:ETS Hearings, Sept 22, 1995.

United States Environmental Protection Agency. Fact sheet: respiratory health effects of passive smoking. U.S. EPA Internet site at http://www.epa.gov/iedweb00/pubs/etsfs.html accessed on 22 january 1998.

———. IAQ publications: sources of information on indoor air quality. U.S. EPA Internet site at http://www.epa.gov/iedweb00/iaq-pubs.html accessed on 22 January 1998; U.S. EPA, Indoor air quality tools for schools:IAQ coordinator's guide. U.S. EPA Internet site at http://www.epa.gov/iedweb00/schools/tfs/guidtoc.html accessed on 14 April 1998; U.S. EPA, Indoor air quality: Basics for schools. U.S. EPA Internet site at http://www.epa.gov/iedweb00/schools/scholkit.html accessed on 22 January 1998; and U.S. EPA, Ventilation and air quality in offices: Fact sheet.U.S. EPA Internet site at http://www.epa.gov/iedweb00/pubs/ventilat.html accessed on 22 January 1998.

———. In contrast, the term building related illness (BRI) is used when symptoms of diagnosable illness are identified an can be attributed directly to airborne building contaminants. Sick building syndrome (SBS): Indoor air facts no. 4 (revised). U.S. EA Internet site at http://www.epa.gov/iedweb00/pubs/sbs.html accessed on 22 January 1998.

———. The inside story: A guide to indoor air quality.

United States Environmental Protection Agency and the United States Consumer Product Safety Commission Office of Radiation and Indoor Air (6604J) EPA Doc 402-K-93-007, A guide to indoor air quality, April 1995.

Van Bronswijk JEMH, Sinha RN. Role of fungi in survival of Dermatophagoides in house-dust environment. *Environ Entomol* 1973;2:142–5.

Van der Heide S, De Monchy JG, De Vries K, Dubois AE, Kauffman HF. Seasonal differences in airway hyperresponsiveness in asthmatic patients: relationship with allergen exposure and sensitization to house dust mites. *Clinical & Experimental Allergy.* 27(6):627–33, 1997 Jun.

Van der Heide S, De Monchy JGR, De Vries K, Bruggnik TM. Seasonal variation in airway hyperresponsiveness and natural exposure to house dust mite allergens in patients with asthma. *J Allergy Clin Immunol* 1994; 93:470–5.

Van Strien RT, Verhoeff AP, Brunekreef B, van Wijnen JH. Mite antigen in house dust: relationship with different housing characteristics in the Netherlands. *Clin Exp Allergy* 1994;24:843–53.

Verhoeff AP, van Strien R, van Wijnen J, Brunekreef B. House dust mite allergen (Der p 1) and respiratory symptoms in children: a case control study. *Clin Exp Allergy* 1994; 49:724–9.

Vervloet D, Charpin D, Haddi E et al. Medication requirements and house-dust mite exposure in mite sensitive asthmatics. *Allergy* 1991; 46:554–8.

Von Essen S MD. Indoor air quality health effects, 1996, 1999.

Wahn U, Lau S, Bergmann R, et al. Indoor allergen exposure is a risk factor for sensitization during the first three years of life. *J Allergy clin Immunol* 1997;99:763–9.

Warner AM, Bjorksten B, Munir AKM, et al. Childhood asthma and exposure to indoor allergens: low mite levels are associated with sensitivity. *Pediatr Allergy Immunol* 1996; 7:61–7. Warner A, Bostrom S, Moller C. Mite fauna in the home and sensitivity to house dust. 1999 54(7):681–90 Jul.

Walshaw MJ, Evans CC. Allergen avoidance in house dust mite sensitive adult asthma. *Q J Med* 1986;58:199–215.

Warner JA, Frederick JM, Bryant TN, Weich C, Raw GJ, Hunter C, Stephen FR, McIntyre DA, Warner JO. Mechanical ventilation and high efficiency vacuum cleaning: A combined strategy of mite and mite allergen reduction in the control of mite-sensitive asthma. *Journal of Allergy & Clinical Immunology* 105(1 Pt 1):75–82, 2000 Jan.

Warner JA, Little SA, Pollock I, Longbottom JL, Warner JO. The influence of exposure to house dust mite, cat, pollen and fungal allergens in the home on sensitization in asthma. *Pediatr Allergy Immunol* 1991;1:79–86.

Weiss ST. Environmental risk factors in childhood asthma. *Clin Exp Allergy* 1998;28(5 Suppl):29–34, 50–1.

Wickens K, Siebers R, Ellis I, Lewis S, Sawyer G, Tohill S, Stone L, Kent R, Kennedy J, Slater T, Crothall A, Trethowen H, Pearce N, Fitzharris P, Crane J. Determinants of house dust mite allergen in homes in Wellington, New Zealand. *Clinical & Experimental Allergy* 27(9):1077–85, 1997 Sep.

Wilkie AT, Ford RPK, Pattemore P, Schluter PJ, Town I, Graham P. Prevalence of childhood asthma symptoms in an industrial suburb of Christchurch. *NZ Med J* 1995; 108:188–90.

Williams LW, Reinfried PS. Eradication of cockroaches does not rapidly reduce cockroach (CR) allergen in vacuumed dust (abstract). *J Allergy Clin Immunol* 1998;101:S156.

Williamson IJ, Martin CJ, McGill G, et al. Damp housing and asthma: a case-control study. *Thorax* 1997; 52:229–34.

Wood R, Laheri A, Eggleston P. The aerodynamic characteristics of cat allergen. *Clin Exp Allergy* 1993;23:733–9.

Wood RA, Chapman MD, Adkinson NF Jr, Eggleston PA. The effect of cat removal on allergen content in household dust samples. *J Allergy Clin Immunol* 1989;83:730–4.

Yunginger JW, Reed CE, O'Connell EJ, Melton LJ III, O'Fallon WM, Silverstein MD. A community-based study of the epidemiology of asthma: incidence rates, 1964-1983. *Am Rev Respir Dis* 1992;146:888–94.

Zeiger RS, Heller S, Mellon MH, et al. Genetic and environmental factors affecting the development of atopy through age 4 in children of atopic parents: a prospective randomized study of food allergen avoidance. *Pediatr Allergy Immunol* 1992; 3:110–27.

Zock JP, Brunekreef B, Hazebrook-Kampschreur AAJM, Roosjen CW. House dust mite allergen in bedroom floor dust and respiratory health of children with asthmatic symptoms. *Eur Respir J* 1994; 7:1254–9.

Zwick H, Popp W, Sertl R, Rauscher H, Wanke T. Allergenic structures in cockroach hypersensitivity. *J Allergy Clin Immunol* 1991;87:626–30.

Notes

Notes

Notes